PROGRAM REVIEW AND EXAMINATION PREPARATION

Surgical Technology
PREP

DATE DUE

Jacqueline R. Bak, MSN, RN, CNOR, CST, RNFA
Director Perioperative Programs
Delaware County Community College
Media, Pennsylvania

Michelle A. Muhammad, CST, AAS
Adjunct Surgical Technologist Instructor
Delaware County Community College
Media, Pennsylvania

Mc
Graw
Hill
Education

New York Chicago San Francisco Athens London Madrid Mexico City
Milan New Delhi Singapore Sydney Toronto

Surgical Technology PREP: Program Review and Examination Preparation

1 2 3 4 5 6 7 8 9 0   LOV   25 24 23 22 21 20 19 18 17

ISBN 978-1-259-58514-2
MHID 1-259-58514-X

Notice

Medicine is an ever-changing science. As new research and clinical experience broaden our knowledge, changes in treatment and drug therapy are required. The authors and the publisher of this work have checked with sources believed to be reliable in their efforts to provide information that is complete and generally in accord with the standards accepted at the time of publication. However, in view of the possibility of human error or changes in medical sciences, neither the authors nor the publisher nor any other party who has been involved in the preparation or publication of this work warrants that the information contained herein is in every respect accurate or complete, and they disclaim all responsibility for any errors or omissions or for the results obtained from use of the information contained in this work. Readers are encouraged to confirm the information contained herein with other sources. For example and in particular, readers are advised to check the product information sheet included in the package of each drug they plan to administer to be certain that the information contained in this work is accurate and that changes have not been made in the recommended dose or in the contraindications for administration. This recommendation is of particular importance in connection with new or infrequently used drugs.

This book was set in Minion Pro by Aptara, Inc.
The editors were Susan Barnes and Peter J. Boyle.
The production supervisor was Richard Ruzycka.
Project management was provided by Dinesh Pokhriyal, Aptara, Inc.
LSC Owensville was printer and binder.

This book was printed on acid-free paper.

Cataloging-in-publication data is on file for this title at the Library of Congress.

To my husband, Larry, for his love and support,
and to my mother, Betty, for her love and constant encouragement.

—*Jacqueline Bak*

To my mother, Mary Lee Rubin, a labor and delivery surgical technologist
for over 40 years in Lafayette, Louisiana

—*Michelle Muhammad.*

Contents

Preface

Surgical Technology PREP is designed to assist you in the review of key concepts and your cumulative knowledge for the certification examination. The book can also assist you in reviewing for a unit exam. As you prepare to take the certification exam, it is important to set up a study schedule and manage your time. Planning is essential to your success. Whether a date is set for the exam or you just have one in mind, use a calendar to map out a plan that allows for a daily routine so that you are not overwhelmed. A target date will keep you motivated and on track.

Concepts to keep in mind when you map out your study plan:

- Review topics and concepts that you find difficult first, allowing appropriate time

- Set up a daily schedule with a target topic/subject matter

- Allow for a minimum of two hours of review each day

- Decide if a study group is appropriate for you

- Schedule practice exams to become comfortable with test questions

- Clarify answers that are not familiar

- Remember to read each question and each answer carefully

- Assess questions that you got incorrect and review that material

- Cramming will only lead to a stressful experience

PART ONE

Fundamental Science

Medical Terminology and Abbreviations

Understanding the language of medicine and specifically surgical procedures and diagnosis begins with medical terminology. Surgical technology students are exposed to this new language from the first day of their education and begin to adapt quickly. Full understanding and review of the common terms will allow the surgical technologist to expand upon their knowledge and increase understanding whether preparing for a unit test or certification exam.

To facilitate understanding and retention of the common medical terminology used in the clinical setting, one must first learn the origins and basis of medical language. Medical terminology language is built from Greek and Latin word parts, eponyms, acronyms, and modern language.

Greek and Latin: terms such as arthritis are built from Greek and Latin word parts.

Eponyms: terms derived from the name of a person, often a physician or scientist who was the first to identify a technique or a condition such as *Alzheimer disease*.

Acronyms: terms formed from the first letters of the words in a phrase that can be spoken as a whole word and usually contain a vowel, such as *laser (light amplification by stimulated emission of radiation)*.

Modern language: terms derived from the English language such as *nuclear medicine scanner*.

In medical terminology, the words are read differently than regular language. Regular language is read from left to right, and medical language is read from right to left.

Example: hepat/itis = hepat (means *liver*), itis (means *inflammation*); this reads *inflammation of the liver.*

All medical terms are divided into two categories:

Terms built from word parts: terms that are composed of Greek and Latin word roots, prefixes, and suffixes and can be translated literally to find their meanings.

Word root: the core of the word; contains the fundamental meaning of the word (Table 1.1).

Example: arthr/itis (*arthr* is the root word meaning *joint*)

Prefix: a word part attached to the beginning of a word root to modify its meaning (Table 1.2).

Example: sub/hepat/ic (*sub* is the prefix that means *under* or *below*)

Suffix: a word part attached to the end of a word root to modify its meaning (Table 1.3).

Example: arthr/itis (*itis* is the suffix meaning *inflammation*).

Combining vowels: a word part, usually an *o*, used to ease pronunciation. Placed to connect two word roots or a word root and a suffix, but not placed to connect a prefix and a word root.

Acronyms or abbreviations can be used for common terms that are used frequently, when this is approved by a facility. An acronym or abbreviation is used when a term is very long, difficult to say or spell, or cumbersome to write out, or if it is a frequently performed procedure. Most health care facilities have a list of approved abbreviations. Acronyms and abbreviations should never be used in the health care setting or in the medical record without first consulting individual health care facility policy.

Some common acronyms and abbreviations you may come across are listed in Table 1.4.

TABLE 1.1	Common Roots		
abdomen/o	abdomen	digit	finger or toe
ablat	take away	dilat	open up, expand, open out
acous	hearing	diverticul	by-road
acumin	to sharpen	ectop	on the outside, displaced
aden/o	gland	embol	plug
adipos/e	fat	eme	to vomit
adnex	connected parts	encephal/o	brain
albin/o	white	enter/o	intestine
alkali	base	enur	urinate
alveol	alveolus, air sac	fasc/i	fascia
amin/o	nitrogen compound	fund/o	fundus
an/o	anus	gall	bile
anastom	join together	gastr/o	stomach
andr/o	male, masculine	gingiv	gums
aneurysm	dilation	glauc	lens opacity, gray
angi/o	blood vessel	gloss/o	tongue
arteri/o	artery	gnosis	knowledge
arteriosus	like an artery	gravid	pregnant
arthr/o	joint	hemat/o	blood
articul	joint	hepar	liver
ascit	fluid in the belly	hepat/o	liver
audi/o	hearing	hyster/o	uterus
auscult	to listen	icterus	jaundice
axill	armpit	ile/o	ileum
balan	glans penis	imperfecta	unfinished
blephar/o	eyelid	inguin	groin
brachi/o	arm	intestine	gut, intestine
buccin	cheek	jugal	throat
capit	head	kel/o	tumor
cardi/o	heart	labi	lip
carp/o	wrist	labyrinth	inner ear
celi	abdomen	lacer	to tear
cephal/o	head	lacrim	tears, tear duct
chete	hair	lingu	tongue
chol/e	bile	lip/o	fat, fatty tissue
col	colon	lith/o	stone
condyl	knuckle	lysis	destruction, to separate
corpus	body	malign	harmful, cancer
cost	rib	mamm/o	breast
cyst/o	bladder, sac, cyst	mast	breast
dacry/o	tears, lacrimal duct	mastic	chew
dermat/o	skin	mediastin/o	mediastinum, middle septum

TABLE 1.1   Common Roots (Continued)

medulla	middle	sigmoid/o	sigmoid colon
pector	chest	sphen	wedge
pelas	skin	splen/o	spleen
pept/i	digest, digestion, amino acid	spondyl	vertebra
pharynx	throat, pharynx	stalsis	to constrict
phleb/o	vein	stern	breastbone, chest
plas	molding, formation	stoma	mouth
pod	foot	tali	ankle bone
proct/o	anus and rectum	tarsus	flat surface
prost/a	prostate	test/o	testicle, testis
ptosis	dropping, falling	thorac/o	chest
pub	pubis	thorax	chest
puer	child	trache/o	trachea
pyel/o	renal pelvis	trauma	wound, injury
pylor	gate, pylorus	ur/o	urinary system
quadr	four	uret	ureter
rect/o	rectum	uvul	uvula
ren	kidney	vag	vagus nerve
retin/o	retina	varus	turn in
rhabd/o	rod-shaped, striated	valgus	turn out
rheumat	a flow, rheumatism	varic/o	dilated, torturous vein
rhin/o	nose	ven/o	vein
rit/u	right	ventr	belly
salping/o	fallopian tube, uterine tube	vesic	sac containing fluid
sarc/o	flesh, sarcoma, muscle	visc/o	sticky
scler/o	hard, white or eye, hardness	viscer	internal organ
scrot	scrotum	xanth	yellow
semin/i	semen	zygot	yoked together

Allan D, Lockyer K. *Medical Language for Modern Health Care*. 3rd ed. New York: McGraw-Hill; 2014.
Booth, K, Stoia, J. *Anatomy, Physiology & Disease for the Health Professions*. 3rd ed. New York: McGraw-Hill; 2013.
Breskin M, Dumith K, Pearsons E, Seeman R. *Medical Dictionary for Allied Health*. New York: McGraw-Hill; 2008.

TABLE 1.2   Common Prefixes

a-, an-	absent, deficient, or without	brady-	slow
ab-	away, from	bucc-	cheek
ad-	toward	carcin-	cancer
adeno-	gland	cardi-	heart
af-	toward	cent-	hundred
angio-	vessel	cephalo-	head
ante-	before	cerebro-	brain
antero-	ahead, in front	cervi-	neck
anti-	against	cheilo-	lips
arthro-	joint	chole-	bile, gall
aur-	ear	chondr-	cartilage
auto-	self	circum-	around
bi-	two	colpo-	vagina
bio-	life	co-, com-, con-	with or together
brachi-	arm	contra-	opposed or against
brachy-	short	cost-	ribs

(continued)

TABLE 1.2   Common Prefixes (Continued)

counter-	against	idio-	self
cranio-	skull	im-	into
cryo-	cold	in-	lacking
crypt-	hidden	infra-	below
cut-	skin	inter-	between
cysto-	bladder, sac	intra-	within
cyto-	cell	ipsi-	same
dactyl-	digits	iso-	equal, same
de-	remove	juxta-	next to
dento-	tooth	kerat-	cornea, keratin
derm-	skin	kil-, kilo-	thousand
dextr-	right	lacri-	tear
di-	twice	lacto-	milk
dia-	across, through	later-	side
diplo-	double	leuko-	white
dis-	apart	litho-	calculi
dorsi-	back	macro-	large
dys-	difficult, painful	mal-	abnormal
e-	out	malacia-	softening
ecto-	external	mast-	breast
ef-	away	mega-	unusually large
en-	in, on	meningo-	membranes covering the CNS central nervous system
endo-	within		
entero-	intestine	meno-	menstrual function
epi-	upon	meso-	middle
erythro-	red	meta-	beyond, change
eu-	good, well	micro-	small
ex-	away from, outside	milli-	one one-thousandth
extra-	beyond, in addition to	mono-	one
fasci-	fibrous tissue	muco-	mucous
fibro-	fibers, threadlike	multi-	many
gastro-	stomach	myco-	fungi
genito-	reproductive organs	myelo-	marrow, spinal canal (cord)
glio-	connective tissue of the central nervous system	myo-	muscle
		necro-	death
gloss-	tongue	neo-	new
glyco-	sugar	nephro-	kidney
gnatho-	jaw	neuro-	nerve
gon-	knee, seed	nocti-	night
gyn-	female	noso-	disease
hem-	blood	ocul-	eye
hemi-	half	oligo-	few, deficient
hepato-	liver	onc-	tumor
hetero-	different	onycho-	nails
histo-	tissue	oo-, ovi-, ovo-	ovum
homeo-	unchanging	oophoro-	ovary
homo-	same	ophthalm-	eye
hydro-	water	ortho-	normal, straight
hyper-	excessive, over	osseo-	bone
hypo-	beneath, deficient, under	oto-	ear
hyster-	uterus	ox-	pertaining to oxygen

TABLE 1.2   Common Prefixes (Continued)

pan-	all	retro-	backward, behind
para-	near	rhino-	nose
path-	disease	salpingo-	tube
ped-	child, foot	sclero-	hard
per-	excessive, through	scolio-	twisted
peri-	around	semi-	partial
phag-	ingest	sept-	poison
phleb-	vein	somato-	body
photo-	light	sono-	sound
pleuro-	membranous lining of thoracic cavity	sta-	stand still
		sten-	narrow
pneumo-	air, lung	sub-	under
pod-	foot	super-	excessive
poly-	many	supra-	above
post-	following, after	sym-	together, with
pre-	before	syn-	together, with
presby-	old	tachy-	rapid
primi-	first	thermo-	heat
pro-	in front of	tox-	poison
procto-	rectum	trach-	windpipe
pseudo-	false	trans-	through, across
psych-	mind	tri-	three
pulmo-	lung	ultra-	excessive
pyelo-	pelvis of kidney	uni-	one
pyo-	pus	vas-	duct, vessel
radio-	emission of radiation	viscero-	internal organs
re-	again, back	xero-	dry
ren-	kidney		

Allan D, Lockyer K. *Medical Language for Modern Health Care*. 3rd ed. New York: McGraw-Hill; 2014.
Booth, K, Stoia, J. *Anatomy, Physiology & Disease for the Health Professions*. 3rd ed. New York: McGraw-Hill; 2013.
Breskin M, Dumith K, Pearsons E, Seeman R. *Medical Dictionary for Allied Health*. New York: McGraw-Hill; 2008.

TABLE 1.3   Common Suffixes

-algia	pain	-emesis	vomiting
-ase	enzyme	-esthesia	sensation
-asthenia	weakness	-ferent	to carry
-atresia	without an opening	-gen	produces, originates
-cele	enlarged cavity, swelling	-glia	connective tissue of the central nervous system
-centesis	removal of fluid via a surgical puncture	-gnosis	knowledge
-cide	cut, kill, destroy	-gram	written or recorded
-clast	break	-graph	writing or recording instrument
-cyte	cell	-graphy	the process of recording
-desis	fusion	-ia	state of
-dynia	pain	-iasis	condition
-ectasis	enlargement or stretching	-ism	state of
-ectomy	surgical removal	-itis	inflammation
-edema	swelling	-lepsy	seizures
-emia	relating to blood or a blood condition	-logist	one who specializes

(continued)

TABLE 1.3   Common Suffixes (Continued)

-lysis	breaking down, destruction, separation	-plegia	paralysis
-malacia	abnormal softening	-pnea	related to breathing
-megaly	large	-ptosis	drooping or prolapsed
-meter	measure	-rrhagia	excessive flow
-oid	like	-rrhaphy	surgical repair of a defect, suture
-ology	study of	-rrhea	flow or discharge
-oma	mass or tumor	-rrhexis	rupture
-opia	vision	-sclerosis	abnormal hardening
-osis	abnormal condition, disease state	-scopy	visual examination
-ostomy	surgically creating a mouth or opening	-soma	body
-otia	ear	-spasm	twitch
-otomy	incision	-stasis	stop or control
-oxia	pertaining to oxygen	-stenosis	abnormal narrowing
-pathy	disease	-taxia	order
-penia	lack of	-tomy	to cut
-pexy	fixation	-tripsy	to crush
-phasia	speak, to say	-trophy	development
-plasty	surgical repair, to shape	-tropic	influencing change
		-uria	related to urination or urine

Allan D, Lockyer K. *Medical Language for Modern Health Care*. 3rd ed. New York: McGraw-Hill; 2014.
Booth, K, Stoia, J. *Anatomy, Physiology & Disease for the Health Professions*. 3rd ed. New York: McGraw-Hill; 2013.
Breskin M, Dumith K, Pearsons E, Seeman R. *Medical Dictionary for Allied Health*. New York: McGraw-Hill; 2008.

TABLE 1.4   Abbreviations

ABG	arterial blood gas	DJD	degenerative joint disease
ACL	anterior cruciate ligament	DNR	do not resuscitate
ADL	activities of daily living	DUB	dysfunctional uterine bleeding
AED	automatic external defibrillator	ECG	electrocardiogram
AIDS	acquired immunodeficiency syndrome	EEG	electroencephalogram
		EKG	electrocardiogram
ASD	atrial septal defect	EMG	electromyogram
ASHD	arteriosclerotic heart disease	ER	emergency room
AVM	arteriovenous malformation	ERCP	endoscopic retrograde cholangiopancreatography
BBB	blood-brain barrier		
BKA	below-the-knee amputation	ESWL	extracorporeal shock wave lithotripsy
BM	bowel movement		
BP	blood pressure	GYN	gynecology
BPH	benign prostatic hypertrophy	HIPAA	Health Insurance Portability and Accountability Act
CABG	coronary artery bypass graft		
CAPD	continuous ambulatory peritoneal dialysis	HIV	human immunodeficiency virus
		H/O	history of
CHF	congestive heart failure	ICD	implantable cardioverter/defibrillator
CJD	Creutzfeldt-Jakob disease		
CPR	cardiopulmonary resuscitation	IUD	intrauterine device
C-section	cesarean section	IVC	inferior vena cava
CSF	cerebrospinal fluid	KUB	x-ray of abdomen to show kidneys, ureters, and bladder
D&C	dilation and curettage		
DIC	disseminated intravascular coagulation	LEEP	loop electrosurgical excision procedure

TABLE 1.4   Abbreviations (Continued)

NKA	no known allergies	ROM	range of motion
NKDA	no known drug allergies	RUQ	right upper quadrant
NPO	nothing by mouth	SC	subcutaneous
OB	obstetrics	SOB	short of breath
OD	right eye	TB	tuberculosis
OS	left eye	THR	total hip replacement
OU	both eyes	TKA	total knee arthroplasty
PDA	patent ductus arteriosus	TMJ	temporomandibular joint
PET	positron emission tomography	TPN	total parenteral nutrition
p.o.	by mouth	TURBT	transurethral resection of bladder tumor
PPH	postpartum hemorrhage	TURP	transurethral resection of the prostate
p.r.n.	when necessary		
q4h	every 4 hours	WNL	within normal limits
q.i.d.	4 times a day		

Allan D, Lockyer K. *Medical Language for Modern Health Care*. 3rd ed. New York: McGraw-Hill; 2014.

Booth, K, Stoia, J. *Anatomy, Physiology & Disease for the Health Professions*. 3rd ed. New York: McGraw-Hill; 2013.

Breskin M, Dumith K, Pearsons E, Seeman R. *Medical Dictionary for Allied Health*. New York: McGraw-Hill; 2008.

Chapter Review Questions

1. Medical terminology language is best described as
   A. Greek and Latin word parts, eponyms, acronyms, and medical language
   B. Greek and Latin words, eponyms, and modern language
   C. Greek and Latin words, acronyms, eponyms, and departments
   D. Greek and Latin word parts, eponyms, acronyms, and modern language

2. Enlargement is indicated by the suffix
   A. -oma
   B. -megaly
   C. -oid
   D. -itis

3. A suffix is
   A. A word part attached to the end of a word root to modify its meaning
   B. A word part attached to the beginning of a word root to modify its meaning
   C. A word part, usually an *o*, used to ease pronunciation
   D. The core of the word

4. *Blepharoplasty* is
   A. Lifting of the eyebrow
   B. Surgical repair of the eyelid
   C. Surgical removal of the eye
   D. The shaping of the head

5. Which one is *not* a root word?
   A. -ectasis
   B. Adipos/e
   C. Balan
   D. Buccin

6. Bilateral salpingo-oophorectomy is
   A. Surgical removal of an ovary
   B. Surgical removal of both fallopian tubes and ovaries
   C. Surgical suspension of both fallopian tubes and ovaries
   D. Surgical removal of both fallopian tubes

7. A patient diagnosed with menorrhagia has
   A. Excessive menstrual flow
   B. Paralysis of menstrual flow
   C. Excessive flow of breathing
   D. Lack of menstrual flow

8. Incision into the bladder is referred to as
   A. Cystoscopy
   B. Chystectomy
   C. Cholecystectomy
   D. Cystotomy

9. The patient is having surgery on the right eye; how is this indicated?
   A. OS
   B. OU
   C. OD
   D. PO

10. Choledochojejunostomy is
    A. A connection between the gallbladder and the stomach
    B. The surgical creation of an opening between the common bile duct and the small intestines
    C. The surgical creation of an opening between the common bile duct and the large intestines
    D. A surgical opening in the gallbladder to the common bile duct, then to the stomach

11. A ureteroscopy is
    A. Removal of a ureter
    B. Endoscopic visualization of the kidney through the ureter
    C. An opening through the skin to drain urine
    D. Visualization of the ureter via fluoroscopy

12. A colostomy is
    A. The examination of the inside of the colon through endoscopy
    B. The surgical removal of the colon
    C. The creation of an opening from the colon to the outside of the body
    D. Inflammation of the colon

13. Pneumonectomy is
    A. The study of breathing
    B. The surgical removal of a lung
    C. The surgical insertion of a chest tube
    D. The surgical removal of a lobe of a lung

14. The surgical technologist is preparing for the surgical procedure when the team is informed that the procedure is cancelled because the patient has bradycardia. Which of the following terms best describes bradycardia?
    A. Rapid heart rate
    B. Irregular heart rate
    C. Slow heart rate
    D. Low hemoglobin

15. The procedure scheduled is a cystoscopy TURP. The surgical technologist knows that TURP when accompanied by cystoscopy usually means
    A. Transurethral resection of polyp
    B. Transurethral renal pelvis
    C. Transurethral radiation of prostate
    D. Transurethral resection of prostate

Answers

1. **D.** Medical terminology language is built from Greek and Latin word parts, eponyms, acronyms, and modern language.
2. **B.** *-megaly* = large.
3. **A.** A suffix is a word part attached to the end of a word root to modify its meaning.
4. **B.** *Blephar/o*= eyelid; *-plasty*= surgical repair, to shape. Meaning: surgical repair of the eyelid.
5. **A.** *-ectasis* is a suffix meaning enlargement or stretching.
6. **B.** *Bilateral* = both sides; *salpingo* = fallopian tube, uterine tube; *oophorectomy* = surgical removal of ovary. Meaning: surgical removal of both fallopian tubes and ovaries.
7. **A.** *Meno-* = menstrual function; *-rrhagia* = excessive flow.
8. **D.** *Cysto* = bladder, sac, *cyst*; -otomy = incision. Meaning: a surgical incision into the urinary bladder.
9. **C.** OD = right eye.
10. **B.** *Choledocho/o* = Common bile duct; *jejun/o* = jejunum (small intestines); *-ostomy* = surgical creation of an opening. Meaning: surgical creation of an opening between the common bile duct and the small intestines (jejunum).
11. **B.** *Uret* = ureter; *-scopy*= visual exam. Visual exam of ureter with a rigid or flexible endoscope.
12. **C.** *Col* = colon; *-ostomy* = surgically creating a mouth or opening.
13. **B.** *Pneumo* = lung; *-ectomy* = surgical removal, excise. Meaning: surgical removal of lung.
14. **C.** *Brady* = slow; *cardia* = heart. Meaning: slow heart rate.
15. **D.** TURP = Transurethral resection of the prostate.

References

Allan D, Lockyer K. *Medical Language for Modern Health Care*. 3rd ed. New York: McGraw-Hill; 2014.

Booth, K, Stoia, J. *Anatomy, Physiology & Disease for the Health Professions*. 3rd ed. New York: McGraw-Hill; 2013.

Breskin M, Dumith K, Pearsons E, Seeman R. *Medical Dictionary for Allied Health*. New York: McGraw-Hill; 2008.

Brooks ML, Brooks DL. *Exploring Medical Language: A Student-Directed Approach*. 8th ed. St. Louis, Mo: Elsevier Mosby; 2011.

2

Anatomy and Physiology

ANATOMICAL TERMINOLOGY

Anatomical Position and Directional Terminology (Figure 2.1)

- ▶ Dorsal: posterior aspect of the body, toward the back
- ▶ Ventral: anterior aspect of the body, toward the front
- ▶ Supine: lying on one's back
- ▶ Prone: lying on one's stomach
- ▶ Sagittal: divides the body into left and right
- ▶ Midsagittal: runs lengthwise down the midline of the body dividing it into equal right and left halves
- ▶ Transverse: (horizontal) divides the body into superior and inferior portions
- ▶ Coronal: (frontal) divides the body into anterior and posterior portions
- ▶ Cephalad: (cranial) superior
- ▶ Caudal: inferior, away from the head
- ▶ Anterior: (ventral) toward the front of the body
- ▶ Posterior: (dorsal) toward the back of the body
- ▶ Medial: toward or closer to the midline
- ▶ Lateral: away from the midline
- ▶ Proximal: closer to the torso or specific part. Example: the hip is proximal to the knee
- ▶ Distal: farther from the torso or a specific part. Example: the knee is distal to the hip

Body Cavities

- ▶ Cranial cavity: contains the brain
- ▶ Spinal cavity: contains the spinal cord
- ▶ Thoracic cavity:
  - » Divided into two pleural cavities (lungs)
  - » Pericardial cavity (heart)
  - » Mediastinum (within the pericardial cavity)
    - • Space between the two lungs laterally, sternum anteriorly, and vertebral column posteriorly
- ▶ Abdominopelvic cavity: divided into superior abdominal cavity and inferior pelvic cavity
  - » Superior abdominal cavity contains:
    - • Stomach
    - • Small and large intestines
    - • Gallbladder
    - • Liver
    - • Spleen
    - • Kidneys
    - • Pancreas

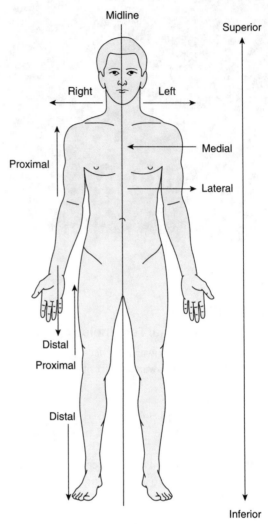

Figure 2.1 Anatomical position.

> » Inferior pelvic cavity
>> • Bladder
>> • Internal reproductive organs
> ▶ Midsternal line: dropped through the center of the sternum. It is a component of the median plane
> ▶ Midclavicular line: dropped through the middle of the clavicle, just medial to the nipple

Tissue Types

▶ Epithelium (epithelial tissue)
> » Lines body cavities, organs, and surfaces
> » Makes up the skin and lines the thoracic and abdominopelvic cavities, esophagus, blood vessels, heart, and stomach
> » Glandular tissue
▶ Skeletal muscle
> » Located throughout the body where voluntary movement takes place
> » Movement of extremities, head, neck, and spine
▶ Cardiac muscle
> » Located in the heart
> » Contract the heart for circulation of blood
▶ Nervous tissue
> » Found in the brain, spinal cord, and nerves
> » Receives, integrates and responds to various internal and external stimuli

▶ Smooth muscle
  » Located in the walls of blood vessels and hollow organs (example: stomach)
  » Maintains blood vessel diameter, controls movement of food through digestive tract
▶ Connective tissue
  » Bone, cartilage, blood, and collagen
  » Transport of oxygen, carbon dioxide, storage of minerals, source of energy, movement

SKIN

▶ The body's first line of defense: a physical barrier
▶ Provides protection, body temperature regulation, and vitamin D production, sensory perception, and excretion
▶ Most common epithelium
▶ A defense mechanism: intact or uncompromised skin protects against bacteria

Composition

▶ Epidermis: top layer most superficial
▶ Dermis: bottom layer, immediately below epidermis
  » Contains all four major tissues
    • Epithelial
    • Connective
    • Muscle
    • Nervous tissue
▶ Subcutaneous (hypodermis): a support layer of tissue
  » Consists mostly of adipose and loose connective tissue
  » Serves as an insulator and cushion
  » Contains blood vessels and nerves

Accessory Organs

▶ Hair/hair follicles: enclosed in follicles, formed from both epidermis and dermis
  » Melanocytes in the follicles produce the pigment giving hair its color
▶ Arrector pili muscles: smooth muscle that connect the hair follicle to papillary layer of dermis
  » Muscles contract, dimpling the skin (goosebumps)
▶ Sebaceous glands: secrete sebum (oil)
  » Found on most areas of the skin except palms of hands and soles of feet
▶ Nails: function to protect the ends of fingers and toes
  » Three main parts
    • Nail body
    • Free edge
    • Cuticle
  » Formed by epithelial cells and hard keratin

Skin Color

▶ Melanin, carotene, and hemoglobin are the three factors that determine skin color
  » Melanin: yellow to brownish black pigment found in some parts of the body such as the skin, retina, and hair
  » Carotene: a yellow pigment found mainly in the stratum corneum and the fat cells of the hypodermis

Rule of Nines (Figure 2.2)

▶ Head: 9% (front and back, 4.5% each)
▶ Right arm: 9% (front and back 4.5% each); left arm: 9% (front and back 4.5% each)
▶ Right leg: 9% (front); left leg: 9% (front)
▶ Right leg: 9% (back); left leg: 9% (back)
▶ Trunk (front): 18%; trunk (back): 18%
▶ Genital area: 1%

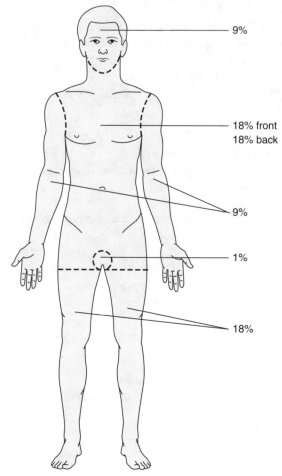

9%

18% front
18% back

9%

1%

18%

Figure 2.2 Rule of nines.

Total body area = 100%.

The rule of nines applies only to adults. For infants a modified rule of nines is used, and for children the Lund and Browder chart is used.

HEAD

Consists of the cranium and the face.

▶ The cranium serves as a protective layer for the brain (8 cranial bones)
▶ The face is composed of several bones (14 facial bones), nerves, muscles, and arteries

Brain

Part of the central nervous system located within the skull. It is responsible for making decisions, solving problems, memory, and much more.

▶ Cerebrum: largest division of the brain. Allows us to think in the present, remember the past, and plan for the future
▶ Diencephalon: contains the thalamus and hypothalamus
  » Thalamus: serves as the relay station for sensory information
  » Hypothalamus: maintains homeostasis by regulating heart rate, blood pressure, and respiration
▶ Brainstem: connects the cerebrum to the spinal cord
  » Midbrain (mesencephalon): controls both visual and auditory reflexes
  » Pons: also regulates respiration
  » Medulla oblongata: controls heart rate, blood pressure, and respiration. It also controls reflexes associated with coughing, sneezing, and vomiting
▶ Cerebellum: coordinates the complex skeletal muscle activity that is needed for body movements. Also coordinates fine motor movements

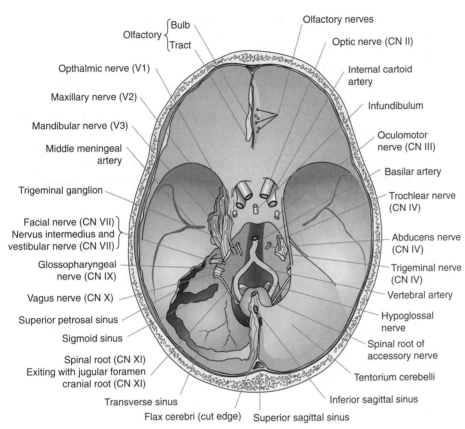

Figure 2.3 Cranial nerves in the interior of the base of the skull. (Reproduced, with permission, from Lalwani A. *Diagnosis & Treatment in Otolaryngology: Head & Neck Surgery.* 3rd ed. New York: McGraw-Hill Education; 2012.)

Cranial Nerves

There are twelve cranial nerves that originate from the brain (Figure 2.3).

▶ I Olfactory: transmits aromas (smells)
▶ II Optic: carries visual information to the brain for interpretation
▶ III Oculomotor: innervates several eye muscles, eye ball, eyelid, and iris
▶ IV Trochlear: innervates the superior oblique muscle of the eye to move the eye down and out. It is the smallest cranial nerve
▶ V Trigeminal: largest of the cranial nerves. Carries sensory information from the surface of the eye, the scalp, facial skin, the lining of the gums, and the palate to the brain for interpretation and also controls mastication (chewing)
▶ VI Abducens: innervates the lateral rectus muscle of the eyeball
▶ VII Facial: innervates the muscles of facial expression as well as the salivary and lacrimal (tear) glands. Also carries sensory information from the tongue
▶ VIII Vestibulocochlear: carries hearing and equilibrium information from the inner ear to the brain for interpretation
▶ IX Glossopharyngeal: carries sensory information from the throat and tongue to the brain for interpretation. Also works with the vagus nerve; responsible for the gag reflex
▶ X Vagus: longest cranial nerve; transmits sensory information from the thoracic and abdominal organs; has motor fibers that innervate the muscles of the throat, stomach, and intestines, and well as the heart
▶ XI Accessory: innervates muscles of the throat, neck, back, and voice box
▶ XII Hypoglossal: responsible for innervating the muscles of the tongue

Eye

A complex organ that processes light to produce images. There are three layers, called tunics.

▶ Fibrous tunic: outer fibrous layer
  » Cornea: helps focus light on the retina

» Sclera: forms the posterior aspect of the outer fibrous tunic; gives structure to the eyeball
▶ Middle layer: uvea (vascular tunic)
» Choroid: vascular component of the eyeball
» Ciliary body: a wedge-shaped thickening in the middle layer of the eyeball; controls the shape of the lens
» Iris: the colored part of the eye that is made up of smooth muscle arranged in both radial and circular orientation
▶ Inner layer
» Retina: nerve cells at the posterior aspect of the retina sense light
• Fovea centralis: sharpest vision area made up of cones (function well in light); rods (function well in dark)
» Optic disk: the blind spot

Ear

Responsible for hearing and, in part, equilibrium
▶ External
» Auricle ("the ear")
» External auditory canal
» Eardrum (tympanic membrane): the boundary between the external and middle ears
▶ Middle
» Ossicles: smallest bones in the body (named because of their shapes)
» Malleus (mallet or hammer)
» Incus (anvil)
» Stapes (stirrup)
▶ Inner
» Labyrinth
• Semicircular canals: three per ear; detect the balance of the body
• Vestibule: also functions in equilibrium
• Cochlea: shaped like a snail's shell and contains hearing receptors

UPPER RESPIRATORY TRACT

▶ Nose/nasal cavity: The nose is the passageway for the entrance and exit of air. It is made up of bone, hyaline cartilage, and adipose tissue covered with skin. The openings of the nose are the nostrils, or external nares. The hairs in the nose assist in preventing debris and unwanted particles from entering the upper respiratory tract via the nares
▶ Oral cavity: The mouth takes in food and reduces its size through mastication. The mouth also starts the process of chemical digestion when saliva, which contains the enzyme amylase, begins to break down carbohydrates
▶ Pharynx: connects the nasal and oral cavities to the esophagus and larynx. It consists of three segments:
» Nasopharynx: from posterior aspect of nasal cavity to soft palate
» Oropharynx: from soft palate to level of hyoid bone. Includes the base of the tongue, lateral/posterior pharyngeal wall, and tonsillar fossae
» Hypopharynx: extends from hyoid bone to inferior aspect of cricoid cartilage and includes pyriform sinuses, postcricoid region, and posterior hypopharyngeal wall
▶ Larynx: forms the air passageway from the hyoid bone to the trachea
» Commonly known as the voice box
» Provides cartilaginous framework for vocal fold and muscle attachment
» Continuous with the laryngopharynx superiorly and the trachea inferiorly
» Provides a patent airway and acts as a switching mechanism to route air and food into the proper channels
▶ Trachea: extends inferiorly from the cricoid cartilage in the midline
» Is halfway between the sternum and vertebral column at the level of the jugular notch

» Sympathetic nerves from T1 to T4 spinal nerves cause airway smooth muscle relaxation and dilation of the airways, parasympathetic innervation of the recurrent laryngeal nerves (CN X) cause airway constriction

SKELETAL SYSTEM

There are 206 bones in the adult skeleton. The function of the skeletal system is for protection and support of the body. The bones in the body acts as a reservoir for over 99% of the calcium in the body. Both white and red blood cells are produced by red bone marrow contained within bone.

▶ Bone is a living connective tissue that contains various types of cells, blood vessels, and nerves
  » Cancellous: spongy bone that has spaces filled with red bone marrow
  » Compact: is denser and has a unique arrangement of cells and canals
    • Osteons: the fundamental unit of compact bone
▶ Bone growth: bone is grown through a process called ossification or osteogenesis
▶ Bone is second only to enamel as the hardest tissue in our body. Bone is a connective tissue, which means that it has a nonliving matrix and living cells
▶ Long bones: classified as such because they are longer than they are wide
  » Femur: the longest and heaviest bone in the body
  » Humerus
  » Tibia and fibula
  » Phalanges: the digits of the hands and feet
▶ Axial skeleton: made up of the skull, ribs, sternum, and vertebra. Consists of 80 bones that lie along the longitudinal axis of the body
  » Facial bone: made up of 14 bones
    • Mandible (1); maxillae (2); zygomatic (2); nasal (2); palatine (2); vomer (1); lacrimal (2); inferior nasal conchae (2)
  » Rib cage: formed by the sternum and 12 pairs of ribs (sternum is made up of three bones)
  » Spinal column: consists of 7 cervical, 12 thoracic, and 5 lumbar vertebrae; a sacrum; and a coccyx
▶ Appendicular skeleton: consists of 126 bones and is made up of the pectoral and pelvic girdles as well as the upper and lower extremities
  » Pectoral girdle: the bones of the shoulders. They attach the upper extremities, or arms, to the axial skeleton
  » Pelvic girdle: consists of the coxal (hip) bones and the lower extremities. The coxal bones attach the legs to the axial skeleton and help protect the pelvic organs
  » Lower extremities: the bones of the lower limb, or leg, include the femur, patella, tibia, fibula, tarsals, metatarsals, and phalanges
  » Joints: are the junctions, or articulations, between bones
    • Fibrous joints: are connected by short connective tissue
    • Synovial joints: the most numerous type of joint in the body, and the most movable. Synovial fluid acts as a lubricant to allow the bones to move easily across each other
▶ Bone fractures:
  » Compound or open fracture: the skin is broken
  » Simple or closed fracture: one where the skin remains intact
  » Greenstick fracture: commonly seen in children, occurs in bones that are not completely ossified so there is a bending rather than a complete breaking of bone
  » Impacted fracture: occurs when the end of the fractured bone is driven into the interior of the other
▶ Bone mass decreases with age. By 30 years of age, this process has already begun in some people. Bone production declines while bone resorption continues at a normal level. Although men lose bone density at the same rate as women after 65 years of age, men typically start with greater bone mass, so in most cases the effects of osteoporosis are not as great in men as in women

ABDOMEN
Abdominal Wall Layers

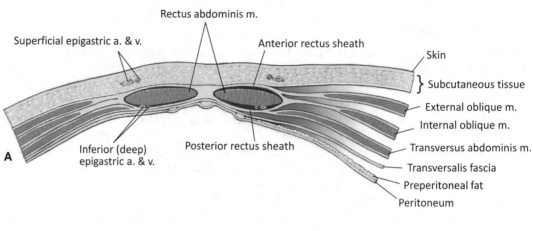

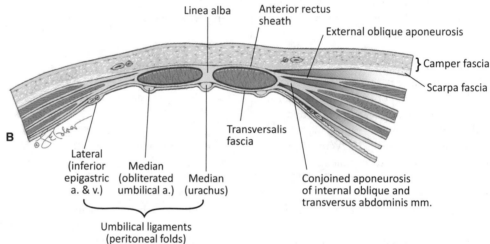

Figure 2.4 Transverse sections of the anterior abdominal wall above (**A**) and below (**B**) the arcuate line. (Reproduced, with permission, from Hoffman B, et al. *Williams Gynecology*. 2nd ed. New York: McGraw-Hill Education; 2012.)

Peritoneum (Figure 2.4)

▶ Visceral peritoneum: innermost layer of the serosa. Secretes serous fluid to prevent organs sticking to other organs
▶ Parietal peritoneum: abdominal lining, secretes serous fluid to prevent sticking to outer layer

DIGESTIVE TRACT

The organs of the gastrointestinal tract (GI tract) and accessory organs are also known as the alimentary canal and extend from the mouth to the anus. It is a muscular tube approximately 26 feet long (tongue to anus) (Figure 2.5).

▶ Esophagus: approximately 10 inches in length, lies posterior to the trachea, descends through the mediastinum in the thoracic cavity and through the diaphragm where it joins the stomach in the abdominal cavity. Uses peristalsis to push food to the stomach
▶ Layers of the GI tract:
  » Mucosa or inner lining (mucous membrane)
  » Submucosa: made up of areolar connective tissue, blood vessels, and nerves
  » Muscularis: composed mostly of smooth muscle, some skeletal muscle
  » Serosa: outermost layer, areolar connective tissue and simple squamous epithelium

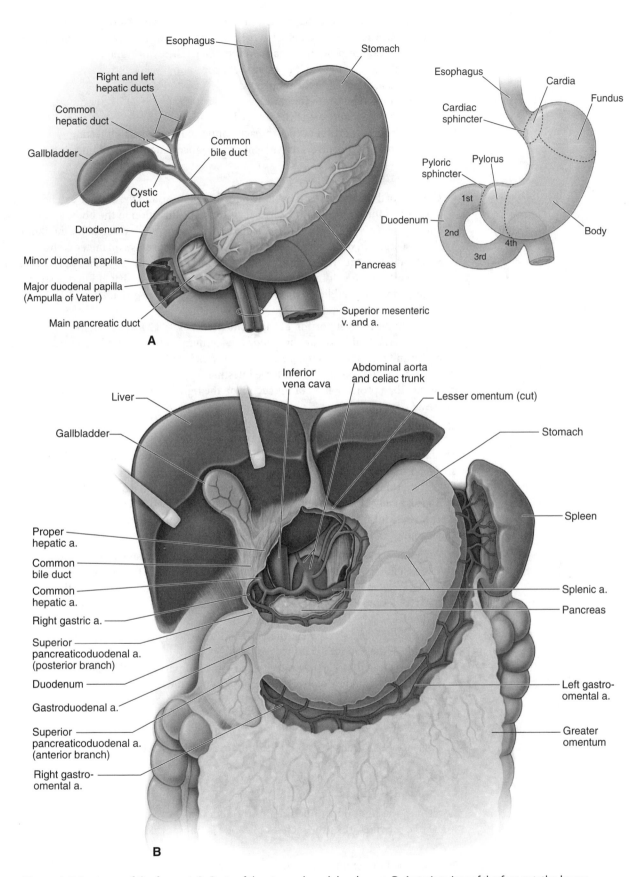

Figure 2.5 Anatomy of the foregut. **A.** Parts of the stomach and duodenum. **B.** Anterior view of the foregut; the lesser omentum is partially removed. (Reproduced, with permission, from Morton DA, Foreman KB, Albertine KH. *Gross Anatomy: The Big Picture*. New York: McGraw-Hill Education; 2011.)

▶ Stomach: lies below the diaphragm in the left upper quadrant of the abdominal cavity. The stomach secretes acid and enzymes; mixing food with secretions to begin the enzymatic digestion or proteins. It has two sphincters; the pyloric and cardiac
   » The stomach is divided into three sections:
      • Cardia: attached to the esophagus
      • Fundus: superior to the cardia
      • Body: the main part of the stomach
▶ Pylorus: narrow portion of the stomach connected to the small intestine
▶ Pylorus sphincter: controls movement of substances into the small intestine

Small Intestine

▶ Consists of three segments; the duodenum, the jejunum, and the ilium. It extends from the stomach to the large intestine, carries out most the digestion in the body, and is responsible for absorbing nutrients. The ileocecal valve joins the last segment, the ilium, with the first segment of the large intestine, the cecum. The average diameter is about 1 inch
   » Duodenum: the first section of the small intestine, about 10 inches in length. At the ampulla of Vater, it receives secretions from the pancreas that aid in digestion
   » Jejunum: the middle portion of the small intestine, approximately 8 feet in length. Begins at the ligament of Treitz
   » Ilium: the longest portion of the small intestines, at 12 feet in length
▶ Mesentery: a fanlike tissue that holds the jejunum and ilium in place in the abdominal cavity and is attached to the posterior abdominal wall
▶ Cecum: the first portion of the large intestine
▶ Appendix: a projection off of the cecum on the right lower quadrant. Contains lymphoid tissue

Colon: The Large Intestine

The large intestine extends from the ileocecal valve to the anus. It averages 5 feet in length and 2.5 inches in diameter. The major function of the large intestine is to absorb water. Other functions include vitamin production and forming and expelling feces.

The large intestine is identified in sections and also identified based on anatomical landmarks. These include the ascending, hepatic flexure, transverse, splenic flexure, descending, and sigmoid colon (Figure 2.6).

▶ Ascending: the portion of the large intestine on the right side of the abdominal cavity. The ascending colon turns at the hepatic flexure, (close to the liver)
▶ Transverse: arising from the ascending colon. Horizontal portion of the large intestine crosses the abdominal cavity and turns at the splenic flexure on the left side of the abdominal cavity (close to the spleen)
▶ Descending: near the spleen, the large intestine becomes the descending colon on the left side of the abdominal cavity
▶ Sigmoid: located in the pelvic cavity, the S-shaped portion of the colon
▶ Rectum: the sigmoid colon straightens to become the rectum
▶ Anal canal/anus: the last portion of the rectum is the anal canal, the opening to the outside of the body (Figure 2.7)

The portal system transports blood from most of the gastrointestinal tract to the liver for metabolic processing before the blood returns to the heart.

Liver (Figure 2.5)

Located in the right upper quadrant of the abdominal cavity. In addition to its numerous metabolic activities, the liver secretes bile. Bile is transported to the gallbladder, where it is stored.

▶ Is attached to the inferior surface of the right dome of the diaphragm via the coronary ligaments
▶ The falciform ligament is a peritoneal structure between the left and right lobes of the liver and the anterior abdominal wall
▶ The liver produces and secretes bile, which emulsifies fat

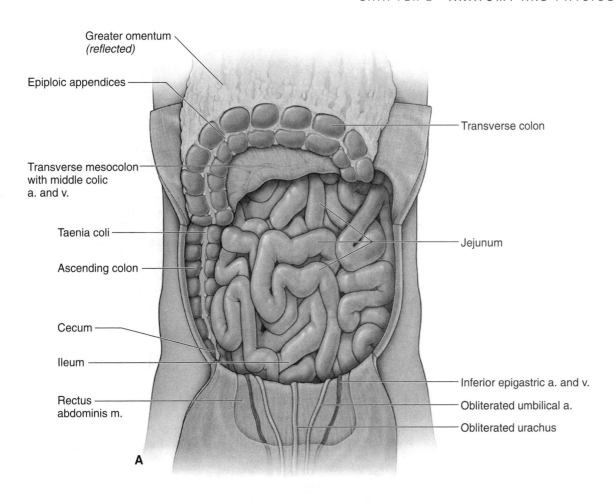

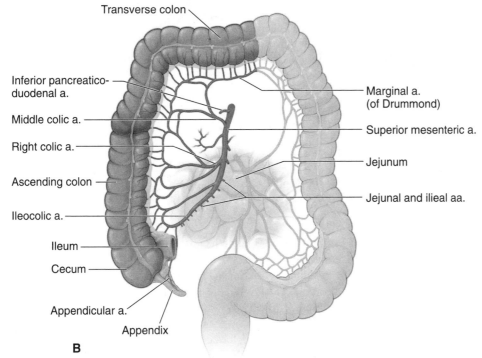

Figure 2.6 Anatomy of the midgut. **A.** Midgut with the greater omentum reflected superiorly and the anterior abdominal wall reflected inferiorly. **B.** Primary blood supply to the midgut is through the superior mesenteric artery. (Reproduced, with permission, from Morton DA, Foreman KB, Albertine KH. *Gross Anatomy: The Big Picture.* New York: McGraw-Hill Education; 2011.)

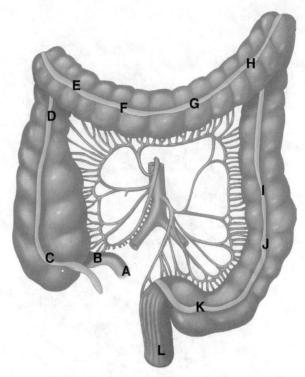

Figure 2.7 Terminology of types of colorectal resections: A→C Ileocecectomy; + A + B→D Ascending colectomy; + A + B→F Right hemicolectomy; + A + B→G Extended right hemicolectomy; + E + F→G + H Transverse colectomy; G→I Left hemicolectomy; F→I Extended left hemicolectomy; J + K Sigmoid colectomy; + A + B→J Subtotal colectomy; + A + B→K Total colectomy; + A + B→L Total proctocolectomy. (Reproduced, with permission, from Fielding LP, Goldberg SM, eds. *Rob & Smith's Operative: Surgery of the Colon, Rectum, and Anus.* London: Elsevier Science Ltd; 1993:349.)

▶ Blood arrives at the liver via two routes:
  » The portal vein: drains from the intestines
  » The hepatic artery

Other functions of the liver include:

▶ Cholesterol metabolism
▶ The urea cycle
▶ Protein production
▶ Clotting factor production
▶ Detoxification
▶ Phagocytosis via the Kupffer cells
▶ Receiving blood from the portal vein and hepatic artery

The liver consists of four lobes:

▶ Right lobe: Positioned to the right of the inferior vena cava and gallbladder
▶ Left lobe: Positioned to the left ligamentum teres
▶ Quadrate lobe: Positioned posterior to the portal triad
▶ Caudate lobe: Positioned anterior to the portal triad

Gallbladder (Figure 2.5)

Lies on the undersurface of the liver, located in the right upper quadrant of the abdominal cavity. The gallbladder stores and concentrates bile secreted by the liver

▶ Bile enters the cystic duct, which joins the common hepatic duct, becoming the common bile duct
▶ The common bile duct and the main pancreatic duct enter the second part of the duodenum at the hepatopancreatic ampulla (of Vater). The sphincter of Oddi surrounds the ampulla and controls the flow of bile and pancreatic digestive enzyme secretions into the duodenum

Pancreas (Figure 2.5)

Retroperitoneal, located behind the stomach. Produces enzymes that chemically digest carbohydrates, proteins, and fats. Pancreatic islets (islets of Langerhans) are found within the pancreas and produce the hormones insulin and glucagon.

The pancreas is divided anatomically into four sections:

▶ Head and neck: found near the curvature of the duodenum
▶ Body and tail: located anterior to the left kidney

Spleen (Figure 2.5)

Located in the left upper quadrant of the abdomen, between the stomach and diaphragm.

▶ The spleen stores blood, produces mononuclear leukocytes, and is responsible for phagocytosis of foreign blood particles
▶ Vascular supply: the pancreas receives blood from branches of both the celiac and superior mesenteric artery. The splenic artery runs along the top margin of the pancreas and supplies the neck, body, and tail of the pancreas through its pancreatic branches, the largest of which is called the greater pancreatic

URINARY SYSTEM

▶ Consists of the kidneys, ureters, bladder and urethra
▶ Contributes to homeostasis
  » Removal of waste product from bloodstream
  » Maintains water and pH balance in body
  » Waste products are excreted in the form of urine

Kidneys

▶ Bean-shaped retroperitoneal organs cushioned by perirenal fat
▶ Located adjacent to vertebrae at T12–2
▶ Right kidney is slightly lower than the left due to liver displacement
▶ The renal artery, renal vein, and ureter enter the kidney at the concave depression known as the hilum
▶ The layers of the kidneys
  » Renal capsule: deepest, protects the kidney from trauma, is continuous with the connective tissue that covers the ureter
  » Middle layer: adipose capsule, protect against trauma and holds the kidney in place
  » Renal fascia: outermost layer, dense, irregular connective tissue that connects anchors the kidney to the abdominal wall
▶ Kidney functions
  » Remove metabolic waste products from blood
  » Helps regulate blood pressure and blood volume (renin)
  » Help regulate pH
  » Participate in the synthesis of vitamin D
  » Involved in gluconeogenesis
▶ Blood supply
  » Renal artery: comes directly off the abdominal aorta, enters the kidney and divides into several segmental arteries (afferent arterioles)
  » Afferent arterioles: branches of the interlobar arcuate arteries that come off the renal artery and supply blood to the nephrons
  » Efferent arteriole: a renal vessel that exits the glomerulus to form a peritubular capillary to form a peritubular capillary
  » Renal vein: formed by the peritubular capillaries and veins that drains into the inferior vena cava
▶ Renal function
  » Nephrons: functional units of the kidney. Made up of a renal corpuscle and tubular system. Filters wastes products from the blood
  » Renal corpuscle: part of the nephron that comprises a glomerulus and Bowman capsule, filters blood
  » Bowman capsule: capsule that surrounds the glomerulus

» Renal tubule: (three parts) proximal convoluted tubule, the loop of Henle, and distal convoluted tubule
» Distal convoluted tubule: merge together to form collecting ducts of urine
» Calyces: transport urine to the renal pelvis
» Renal pelvis: cavity in the center of the kidney where the mayor calyces open

Bladder and Ureters

Ureters: long, muscular tubes that drain urine from the kidneys. Urine is carried through the ureters to the bladder via peristalsis. Enter the bladder at the trigone
   Bladder: located in the pelvic cavity just below the symphysis pubis.

▶ Interior is lined with mucosal folds called rugae that allow for expansion
▶ Approximately 800 mL urine capacity
▶ Apex: the top of the bladder. Located at the top of the symphysis pubis
▶ Base: located inferiorly and posteriorly. The ureters enter the bladder at each of the superior corners of the base of the bladder
▶ Trigone: an internal landmark. The triangular area inside the bladder between the openings of the ureters
▶ Neck: most inferior portion of the bladder, surrounds the origin of the urethra
▶ Internal urethral sphincter: smooth muscle that involuntarily contracts or relaxes, regulating the emptying of the bladder
▶ External urethral sphincter: voluntarily opens and closes the urethra to void urine
▶ Layers of the Bladder:
   » Mucosa (inner most layer) transitional epithelium
   » Muscular layer (middle layer) detrusor muscle—responsible for contraction to push urine from bladder through urethra (micturition)
   » Superficial layer (connective tissue)

Urethra

A tube that expels urine from the bladder to outside the body.

▶ Female urethra 4 inches in length
▶ Male urethra 8 inches in length

REPRODUCTIVE SYSTEM

Male Reproductive System

▶ The male external reproductive organs are the scrotum, testes, and penis
   » Scrotum: the pouch of skin that holds the testes away from the rest of the body, keeping their temperature about one degree lower than that of the core of the body, which is necessary for the sperm to live
   » Testes: the primary organs of the male reproductive system. They produce the sex cells (sperm) of the male and also produce the male hormone testosterone
   » Penis: a highly vascularized cylindrical organ that propels urine and semen outside the body. The shaft, or body, of the penis contains specialized erectile tissue that surrounds the urethra and runs the length of the penis
      • Glans penis is the end of the penis that enlarges into a cone-shaped structure. A piece of skin (if the male has not been circumcised) called the prepuce or foreskin covers the glans penis
      • The function of the penis is to deliver sperm to the female reproductive tract and is also functions during urination by draining urine from the bladder
▶ Internal male reproductive structures
   » Epididymis: where sperm is kept during the maturing phase of growth
   » Vas deferens: carry sperm cells from each epididymis to the urethra
   » Accessory sex glands
      • Seminal vesicle: saclike organs that secrete an alkaline fluid rich in sugars and prostaglandins and make up 60% of the semen volume. The sugars are used by sperm for energy

- Prostate gland: surrounds the proximal portion of the urethra. It produces a milky, alkaline fluid that is secreted into the urethra just before ejaculation. This fluid helps protect the sperm when they enter the more acidic environment of the female vagina. This fluid makes up approximately 40% of semen volume
- Bulbourethral glands: inferior to the prostate gland. They produce a mucus-like fluid that is secreted before ejaculation into the urethra. This fluid lubricates the end of the penis in preparation for sexual intercourse
- Semen: a mixture of sperm cells and fluids from the seminal vesicles, prostate gland, and bulbourethral glands. This mixture is alkaline to counteract the acidic environment of the vagina and contains nutrients and prostaglandins. A normal sperm count is considered to be more than 80 million per milliliter

Female Reproductive System

Nurtures a developing offspring. It produces a number of important hormones before and during the reproductive years

► External female reproductive Structures
  » Vulva
    - Mons pubis: fatty area that overlies the pubic symphysis
    - Labia majora: rounded folds of adipose tissue and skin that protect the other external female reproductive organs (covered in pubic hair)
    - Labia minora: folds of skin between the labia majora
    - Clitoris: anterior to the urethral meatus. It contains the female erectile tissue and is rich in sensory nerves
    - Urethral meatus: the opening in the urethra through which urine is secreted
    - Vaginal orifice: the opening to the vagina
    - Bartholin glands: on either side of the vaginal orifice and secrete mucus for lubrication
    - Perineum: the area between the vagina and anus
  » Mammary glands: secretion of milk for newborn offspring and located beneath the skin of the chest
► Internal female reproductive structures
  » Ovaries: The primary sex organs of the female. They produce female sex cells (ova) and also produce estrogen and progesterone, the female hormones
    - Oogenesis: the process of ovum formation
  » Fallopian tube (oviduct): One opens near each ovary; other end connects to the uterus. Its function is to catch an ovum and propel the ovum toward the uterus using peristalsis and the sweeping motions of cilia. This is where fertilization occurs
  » Uterus: a hollow, muscular organ that receives a developing embryo and sustains its development
    - Fundus: upper domed portion of the uterus
    - Body: the main portion
    - Cervix: lower narrow portion that extends into the vagina. The opening of the cervix is called the cervical orifice, or os
  » Vagina: a tubular, muscular organ that extends from the uterus to outside the body
  » Broad ligament: the wide fold of peritoneum that connects the sides of the uterus to the walls and floor of the pelvis
  » Round ligament: this ligament is responsible for maintaining the anteversion of the uterus (a position where the fundus of the uterus is turned forward at the junction of cervix and vagina) during pregnancy

Chapter Review Questions

1. Using the rule of nines, what is the total percentage for a patient who has suffered burns to one leg (circumferential), one arm (circumferential), and the anterior trunk?
   A. 18%
   B. 27%
   C 36%
   D. 45%

2. The term *proximal* refers to
   A. away from the head.
   B. being comparatively closer to the midline.
   C. a structure being closer to the trunk or a specified part.
   D. relatively farther from the midline.

3. Which cranial nerve is responsible for transmitting impulses that move the eyes?
   A. Abducens (VI)
   B. Vestibulocochlear (VIII)
   C. Olfactory (I)
   D. Optic (II)

4. Where are the kidneys located?
   A. Peritoneal cavity
   B. Thoracic cavity
   C. Pelvic cavity
   D. Retroperitoneal cavity

5. What are the primary organs of the male reproductive system?
   A. The seminiferous tubules
   B. The penis
   C. The testes
   D. The scrotum

6. Where does fertilization of the female ovum occur?
   A. Ovary
   B. Fallopian tube
   C. Fundus of uterus
   D. Cervix

7. Where would you find smooth muscles?
   A. Wall of the heart
   B. Walls of hollow organs, blood vessels, and iris
   C. Attached to bones and skin of the face
   D. None of the above

8. What is the functional unit(s) of the kidney?
   A. Nephron
   B. Bowman capsule
   C. Calyces
   D. Renal pelvis

9. Which of the following best describes the function of the gallbladder?
   A. Secrete bile
   B. Convert bile
   C. Store bile
   D. Excrete stones

10. **What portion of the large intestine is located in the pelvic cavity and is S-shaped?**
    A. Ascending colon
    B. Descending colon
    C. Rectum
    D. Sigmoid colon

11. **Which ligament is used as an anatomical landmark to identify the end of the duodenum?**
    A. Cruciate ligament
    B. Round ligament
    C. Ligament of Treitz
    D. Umbilical ligament

12. **The layers of the gastrointestinal tract from the inner to outer layers in order are**
    A. submucosa, muscularis, serosa, mucosa.
    B. mucosa, submucosa, muscularis, serosa.
    C. muscularis, serosa, mucosa, submucosa.
    D. serosa, mucosa, submucosa, muscularis.

13. **An open fracture is referred to as a(n)**
    A. simple fracture.
    B. greenstick fracture.
    C. impacted fracture.
    D. compound fracture.

14. **The first portion of the large intestine is the**
    A. duodenum.
    B. cecum.
    C. ilium.
    D. jejunum.

15. **The major function of the large intestine is to**
    A. absorb bile.
    B. absorb nutrients.
    C. absorb water.
    D. absorb digestive enzymes.

16. **The _____ colon is on the right side of the body and makes a turn at the _____ flexure.**
    A. descending; splenic
    B. ascending; hepatic
    C. transverse; splenic
    D. sigmoid; rectal

17. **This internal landmark of the bladder is where the ureters enter the bladder.**
    A. The trigone
    B. The dome
    C. The base
    D. The apex

18. **The two sphincters of the stomach are the**
    A. fundal and esophageal.
    B. hepatic and cardiac.
    C. pyloric and cardiac.
    D. gastric and pyloric.

19. The _____ forms the air passageway from the hyoid bone to the trachea.
    A. larynx
    B. pharynx
    C. oropharynx
    D. nasopharynx

20. **The primary function of the liver is to**
    A. secrete insulin.
    B. produce glucagon.
    C. secrete bile.
    D. assist in digestion.

Answers

1. **D.** 45%. One leg circumferentially = 18%, one arm circumferentially = 9%, and anterior trunk = 18%
2. **C.** A structure being closer to the trunk or a specified part
3. **A.** Abducens (VI)
4. **D.** Retroperitoneal cavity
5. **C.** Testes
6. **B.** Fallopian tube
7. **B.** Walls of hollow organs, blood vessels and iris
8. **A.** The nephron is the functional unit
9. **C.** The gallbladder stores bile
10. **D.** Sigmoid colon
11. **C.** Ligament of Treitz
12. **A.** Mucosa, submucosa, muscularis, serosa
13. **D.** Compound fracture
14. **B.** Cecum
15. **C.** Absorbing water is the main function of the large intestine
16. **B.** Ascending; hepatic
17. **C.** The base
18. **C.** Pyloric and cardiac
19. **A.** Larynx
20. **C.** Secrete bile

References

Booth K, Wyman T, Stoia V. *Anatomy, Physiology, and Disease for Health Professionals.* 3rd ed. New York: McGraw-Hill Education; 2012.

Morton DA, Foreman K, Albertine KH. Chapter 9. Foregut. In Morton DA, Foreman K, Albertine KH, eds. *Gross Anatomy: The Big Picture.* New York: McGraw-Hill Education; 2011. Retrieved April 9, 2016, from http://accessmedicine.mhmedical.com/content.aspx?bookid=381&Sectionid=40140016.

Morton DA, Foreman K, Albertine KH. Chapter 28. Larynx. In Morton DA, Foreman K, Albertine KH, eds. *Gross Anatomy: The Big Picture.* New York: McGraw-Hill Education; 2011. Retrieved July 29, 2016, from http://accessmedicine.mhmedical.com/content.aspx?bookid=381&Sectionid=40140037.

Weinberger PM, Terris DJ. Otolaryngology: head & neck surgery. In: Doherty GM, ed. *CURRENT Diagnosis & Treatment: Surgery.* 14th ed. New York: McGraw-Hill Education; 2015. Retrieved July 29, 2016, from http://accessmedicine.mhmedical.com/content.aspx?bookid=1202&Sectionid=71517698.

3

Microbiology

Microbiology is a specialized area of biology that deals with living things ordinarily too small to be seen without magnification. Such microscopic organisms are collectively referred to as microorganisms, microbes, or several other terms depending on the kind of microbe or the purpose. In surgery it is important to know about the microbes in the surgical environment so they can be properly removed to create a sterile environment.

GROUPS OF MICROBES

► Bacteria: Has no true nucleus. Bacteria function as independent single-celled, or unicellular, organisms. Each individual bacterial cell is fully capable of carrying out all necessary life activities, such as reproduction, metabolism, and nutrient processing, unlike the more specialized cells of a multicellular organism. One of the most important ways to describe bacteria is by their shape and arrangement. Gram stains are a staining technique that delineates two generally different groups of bacteria. The technique of Hans Christian Gram consisted of timed, sequential applications of crystal violet (the primary dye), Gram iodine (the mordant), an alcohol rinse (decolorizer), and a contrasting counterstain. Bacteria that stain purple are called gram-positive, and those that stain red are called gram-negative. This century-old staining method remains the universal basis for bacterial classification and identification. This is a practical aid in diagnosing infection and in guiding drug treatment
  » External appendages
    • Flagella, pili, fimbriae
  » Cell envelope
    • Cell wall
    • Cytoplasmic membrane
  » Internal
    • Cytoplasm
    • Ribosomes
    • Inclusions
    • Nucleoid/chromosome
    • Cytoskeleton
    • Endospore
    • Plasmid
    • Microcompartments
► Archaea: Simple, single-celled organisms that share many bacterial characteristics. This organism has a different ribosomal RNA sequence than is found in bacteria and have entirely unique sequences in their rRNA. Archaea are the most primitive of all life forms and are most closely related to the first cells that originated on the earth 4 billion years ago. They are often called extremophiles, meaning that they "love" extreme conditions in the environment. This kind of microbe must be dealt with extremely to create a sterile

TABLE 3.1   Major Fungal Infections of Humans

Degree of Tissue Involvement and Area Affected	Name of Infection	Name of Causative Fungus
Superficial (not deeply invasive)		
Outer epidermis	Tinea versicolor	*Malassezia furfur*
Epidermis, hair, and dermis	Dermatophytosis, also called tinea or ringworm of the scalp, body, feet (athlete's foot), toenails	*Microsporum, Trichophyton*, and *Epidermophyton*
Mucous membranes, skin, nails	Candidiasis, or yeast infection	*Candida albicans*
Systemic (deep; organism enters lungs; can invade other organs)		
Lung	Coccidioidomycosis (San Joaquin Valley fever)	*Coccidioides immitis*
	North American blastomycosis (Chicago disease)	*Blastomyces dermatitidis*
	Histoplasmosis (Ohio Valley fever)	*Histoplasma capsulatum*
	Cryptococcosis	*Cryptococcus neoformans*
Lung, skin	Paracoccidioidomycosis (South American blastomycosis)	*Paracoccidioides brasiliensis*

environment. Archaea are not just environmental microbes. They have been isolated from human tissues such as the colon, mouth, and vagina. Recently, an association was found between the degree of severity of periodontal disease and the presence of archaeal RNA sequences in the gingiva, suggesting—but not proving—that Archaea may be capable of causing human disease

▶ Fungi: All fungi are heterotrophic (organisms that rely on organic compounds for its carbon and energy needs). Fungi can also be parasites on the bodies of living animals or plants, although very few fungi absolutely require a living host. They are often found in nutritionally poor or adverse environments. During the development of a fungal colony, the vegetative hyphae give rise to structures called reproductive, or fertile, hyphae, which branch off a vegetative mycelium. These hyphae are responsible for the production of fungal reproductive bodies called spores (Table 3.1)

▶ Protozoa: means "first animals." There are about 12,000 species of protozoa. Although single-celled, protozoa have startling properties when it comes to movement, feeding, and behavior. Although most members of this group are harmless, free-living inhabitants of water and soil, a few species are parasites collectively responsible for hundreds of millions of infections of humans (Table 3.2)

TABLE 3.2   Major Pathogenic Protozoa

Protozoan	Disease	Reservoir/Source
Amoeboid Protozoa (Sarcodina)		
Entamoeba histolytica	Amoebiasis (intestinal and other symptoms)	Humans, water, and food
Naegleria, Acanthamoeba	Brain infection	Water
Ciliated Protozoa (Ciliophora)		
Balantidium coli	Balantidiosis (intestinal and other symptoms)	Pigs, cattle
Flagellated Protozoa (Mastigophora)		
Giardia lamblia	Giardiasis (intestinal distress)	Animals, water, and food
Trichomonas vaginalis	Trichomoniasis (vaginal symptoms)	Human
Trypanosoma brucei, T. cruzi	Trypanosomiasis (intestinal distress and widespread organ damage)	Animals, vector-borne
Leishmania donovani, L. tropica, L. brasiliensis	Leishmaniasis (either skin lesions or widespread involvement of internal organs)	Animals, vector-borne
Apicomplexan Protozoa (Sporozoa)		
Plasmodium vivax, P. falciparum, P. malariae	Malaria (cardiovascular and other symptoms)	Human, vector-borne
Toxoplasma gondii	Toxoplasmosis (flulike illness or silent infection)	Animals, vector-borne
Cryptosporidium	Cryptosporidiosis (intestinal and other symptoms)	Waver, food
Cyclospora cayetanensis	Cyclosporiasis (intestinal and other symptoms)	Water, fresh produce

► Helminthes: From the Greek word meaning "worm." Adult specimens are usually large enough to be seen with the naked eye, and they range from the longest tapeworms, measuring up to about 25 m in length, to roundworms less than 1 mm in length. Sources for human infection are contaminated food, soil, and water or infected animals; routes of infection are by oral intake or penetration of unbroken skin

  » Flat worms: phylum Platyhelminthes; have a very thin, often segmented body plan

  » Round worms: phylum Aschelminthes (nematodes); have an elongated, cylindrical, unsegmented body

► Viruses: Viruses are a unique group of biological entities known to infect every type of cell, including bacteria, algae, fungi, protozoa, plants, and animals. They have been known to infect other cells and sometimes influence their genetic makeup. They have shaped the way cells, tissues, bacteria, plants, and animals have evolved to their present forms. Viruses cannot multiply unless they invade a specific host cell and instruct its genetic and metabolic machinery to make and release quantities of new viruses

► Algae: They are photosynthetic, plantlike organisms that generally lack the complex structure of plants; they may be single-celled or multicellular and inhabit diverse habitats such as marine and freshwater environments, glaciers, and hot springs

THE PROCESS OF INFECTION

► Portals of entry: To initiate an infection, a microbe enters the tissues of the body by a characteristic route, the portal of entry, usually the skin or a mucous membrane. The source of the infectious agent can be exogenous, originating from a source outside the body (the environment or another person or animal) or endogenous, already existing on or in the body (normal biota or a previously silent infection)

  » Skin

    • *Staphylococcus aureus*, *Streptococcus pyogenes*, *Clostridium tetani*

    • Herpes simplex (type 1)

    • Helminth worms

    • Viruses, rickettsia, protozoa (e.g., malaria, West Nile virus)

    • *Haemophilus aegyptius*, *Chlamydia trachomatis*, *Neisseria gonorrhoeae*

  » Gastrointestinal tract

    • *Salmonella*, *Shigella*, *Vibrio*, *Escherichia coli*, poliovirus, hepatitis A, echovirus, rotavirus, enteric protozoans (*Giardia lamblia*, *Entamoeba histolytica*)

  » Respiratory tract

    • Bacteria causing meningitis, influenza, measles, mumps, rubella, chickenpox, common cold, *Streptococcus pneumoniae*, *Klebsiella*, *Mycoplasma*, *Cryptococcus*, *Pneumocystis*, *Mycobacterium tuberculosis*, *Histoplasma*

  » Urogenital tract

    • Human immunodeficiency virus (HIV), *Trichomonas*, hepatitis B, syphilis, *Treponema pallidum*, *Neisseria gonorrhoeae*, *Chlamydia trachomatis*, herpes, genital warts

► Becoming established: attaching to the host

  » Adhesion is a process by which microbes gain a more stable foothold on host tissues. There are many different methods by which microbes can attach themselves. Firm attachment to host tissues is almost always a prerequisite for causing diseases, because the body has so many mechanisms for flushing microbes and foreign materials from its tissues

► Becoming established: surviving host defenses

  » Microbes that are not established in a normal biota relationship in a particular body site in a host are likely to encounter resistance from host defenses when first entering, especially from certain white blood cells called phagocytes. These cells ordinarily engulf and destroy pathogens by means of enzymes and antimicrobial chemicals

► Causing disease

  » Virulence factors are structures or capabilities that allow a pathogen to cause infection in a host. From a microbe's perspective, they are simply adaptations it uses to invade and establish itself in the host. The effects of a pathogen's virulence factors on tissues vary greatly. Cold viruses, for example, invade and multiply but cause relatively little damage to their host. At the other end of the spectrum, pathogens such as

Clostridium tetani or HIV severely damage or kill their host. There are three major ways that microorganisms damage their host:
- Directly through the action of enzymes
- Directly through the action of toxins (both endotoxin and exotoxins)
- Indirectly by inducing the host's defenses to respond excessively or inappropriately

» Signs and symptoms of inflammation
- Signs: edema, accumulation of fluid in an afflicted tissue, granulomas and abscesses, walled-off collections of inflammatory cells and microbes in the tissues; and lymphadenitis, swollen lymph nodes
- Symptoms: fever, pain, soreness, and swelling

▶ Vacating the host: portals of exit
» In most cases, the pathogens are shed or released from the body through secretion, excretion, discharge, or sloughed tissue
- Incubation period: the time from initial contact with the infectious agent to the appearance of the first symptoms
- Prodromal stage: short period (1–2 days)
- Period of invasion: the pathogen multiplies at high levels, exhibits its greatest virulence, and becomes well established in its target tissue
- Convalescent period: the patient's strength and health gradually return because of the healing nature of the immune response

▶ Infectious diseases that are acquired or developed during a stay at a hospital or health care facility are known as health care–associated or nosocomial infections. The most common health care–associated infections involve the urinary tract (bladder infections from Foley catheters), the respiratory tract (pneumonia from lack of movement), and surgical incisions (surgical site infections from break in sterile technique)

DISEASES AFFECTING BODY SYSTEMS

▶ Skin and eyes:
» Microbes that do live on the skin surface as normal biota must be capable of living in the dry, salty conditions they find there. Microbes are relatively sparsely distributed over dry, flat areas of the body, such as on the back, but they can grow into dense populations in moist areas and skin folds, such as the underarm and groin areas. The normal microbiota also live in the protected environment of the hair follicles and glandular ducts
- Methicillin-resistant *Staphylococcus aureus* (MRSA)
- *Staphylococcus aureus*: remains viable after months of air drying and resists the effect of many disinfectants and antibiotics
» Conjunctiva of the eye: The eye's best defense is the film of tears, which consists of an aqueous fluid, oil, and mucus. Inflammation does not occur in the eye as readily as it does elsewhere in the body
- *Neisseria*: species that can live on the surface of the eye
- Diseases:
  - Conjunctivitis: pink eye
  - Keratitis: usual cause of herpetic keratitis is a "misdirected" reactivation of (oral) herpes simplex virus type I (KSV-1)

▶ Nervous system:
» It is still believed that there is no normal biota in either the central nervous system (CNS) or peripheral nervous system (PNS), and that finding microorganisms of any type in these tissues represents a deviation from the healthy state
- Meningitis: an inflammation of the meninges
- Neonatal meningitis: is almost always a result of infection transmitted by the mother, either in utero or (more frequently) during passage through the birth canal
- Poliomyelitis: an acute enteroviral infection of the spinal cord that can cause neuromuscular paralysis, often in small children
- Meningoencephalitis: disease in both the meninges and brain
- Acute encephalitis: inflammation of the brain

- Subacute encephalitis: most commonly causes by the protozoan *Toxoplasma* (infection in the fetus and in immunodeficient people)
- Rabies: a slow, progressive zoonotic disease characterized by a fatal encephalitis
- Tetanus: lockjaw
- Botulism: caused by an exotoxin associated with eating poorly preserved foods

▶ Cardiovascular and lymphatic systems
  » The cardiovascular system is the pipeline of the body. It is composed of the blood vessels, which carry blood to and from all regions of the body, and the heart, which pumps the blood. The cardiovascular system provides tissues with oxygen and nutrients and carries away carbon dioxide and waste products, delivering them to the appropriate organs for removal. The lymphatic system is a major source of immune cells and fluids and serves as a one-way passage, returning fluid from the tissues to the cardiovascular system
    - Malaria: has been one of the greatest afflictions, in the same rank as bubonic plague, influenza, and tuberculosis. *Mal*, "bad" and *aria*, "air"
    - HIV infection and AIDS: Acquired immunodeficiency syndrome (AIDS) is the result of an HIV infection if T-cell levels drop too low
    - Endocarditis: an inflammation of the endocardium, or inner lining of the heart. Usually it involves the mitral or aortic valve
    - Septicemia: occurs when organisms are actively multiplying in the blood
    - Plague: infection by the bacterium causing plagues
      - Pneumonic; bubonic; septicemic; purpura
    - Tularemia: sometimes called "rabbit fever"
    - Lyme disease: often evolves into a slowly progressive syndrome that mimics neuromuscular and rheumatoid conditions
    - Infectious mononucleosis: a lymphatic system disease, which is often simply called "mono" or the "kissing disease"
    - Nonhemorrhagic fever diseases: syndromes characterized by high fever but without the capillary fragility that leads to hemorrhagic symptoms
    - Q fever: the Q stands for "query"
    - Rocky Mountain spotted fever (RMSF): caused by a bacterium called *Rickettsia rickettsii* transmitted by hard ticks such as the wood tick, the American dog tick, and the Lone Star tick
    - Chagas disease: "the American trypanosomiasis." Has been called "the new AIDS of the Americas" because it has a long incubation time and is very difficult to cure
    - Anthrax: causes disease in the lungs and in the skin and multiplies in large numbers in the blood

▶ Respiratory systems:
  » The respiratory tract is the most common place for infectious agents to gain access to the body. We breathe 24 hours a day, and anything in the air we breathe passes at least temporarily into this organ system
    - Pharyngitis: inflammation of the throat
    - The common cold: caused by one of more than 200 different kinds of viruses
    - Sinusitis: called a sinus infection, this inflammatory condition of any of the four pairs of sinuses in the skull can actually be caused by allergy, infections, or simply by structural problems such as narrow passageways or a deviated nasal septum
    - Acute otitis media (ear infection): upper respiratory tract infections lead to inflammation of the eustachian tubes and the buildup of fluid in the middle ear, which can lead to bacterial multiplication in those fluids
    - Diphtheria: caused by a non–endospore-forming, gram-positive club-shaped bacterium
    - Influenza: the "flu"; commonly acquired during the winter months and tends to evolve into a different strain on a regular seasonal span
    - Whooping cough (pertussis): there are three stages to this disease
      - Catarrhal phase: begins when bacteria present in the respiratory tract cause what appear to be cold symptoms, most notably a runny nose
      - Paroxysmal phase: characterized by severe and uncontrollable coughing

- Convalescent phase: the time when number of bacteria are decreasing and no longer cause ongoing symptoms
- Respiratory syncytial virus (RSV) infection: infects the respiratory tract and produces giant multinucleated cells; children 6 months of age or younger, as well as premature babies, are especially susceptible to serious disease caused by this virus
- Tuberculosis (TB): called "Captain of the Men of Death" and "White Plague"; chronic bacterial infection of the lungs or other tissues caused by *Mycobacterium tuberculosis* organisms
- Pneumonia: an inflammatory condition of the lung in which fluid fills the alveoli

▶ Gastrointestinal (GI) tract
  » The GI tract has a very heavy load of microorganisms, and it encounters millions of new ones every day. Because of this, defenses against infection are extremely important. All intestinal surfaces are coated with a layer of mucus, which confers mechanical protection
  - Acute diarrhea: defined as three or more loose stools in a 24-hour period
  - Food poisoning: when a patient presents with severe nausea and frequent vomiting accompanied by diarrhea, and reports that companions with whom he or she shared a recent meal (within the last 1 to 6 hours) are suffering the same fate, food poisoning should be suspected
  - Tooth and gum infections: if left undisturbed, the biofilm structure eventually contains anaerobic bacteria that can result in breakdown of hard tooth structure (the dentition) due to the production of acid by certain oral streptococci in the biofilm
  - Dental caries (tooth decay): involves the dissolution of solid tooth surface due to the metabolic action of bacteria
  - Periodontal diseases: most kinds are due to bacterial colonization and varying degrees of inflammation that occur in response to gingival damage
  - Mumps: Old English for "lump" or "bump." Mildly epidemic illness associated with painful swelling at the angle of the jaw
  - Gastritis and gastric ulcers: experienced as sharp or burning pain emanating from the abdomen. Gastric or peptic ulcers are actual lesions in the mucosa of the stomach or in the uppermost portion of the small intestines
  - Hepatitis: an inflammatory disease marked by necrosis of hepatocytes and a mononuclear response that swells and disrupts the liver architecture
  - Hepatitis B virus (and hepatitis D): Hepatitis B virus is an enveloped DNA virus in the family Hepadnaviridae
  - Helminthic infections: intestinal distress as the primary symptom. Both tapeworms and roundworms can infect the intestinal tract in such a way as to cause primary symptoms there
  - Helminthic infections: intestinal distress accompanied by migratory symptoms: a diverse group of helminthes enter the body as larvae or eggs, mature to the worm stage in the intestine, and then migrate into the circulatory and lymphatic systems, then to the heart, lungs, migrate up to the respiratory tree to the throat, and are swallowed, then take up residence in the intestinal tract
  - Cysticercosis: a tapeworm that attach to the intestine. Infection caused by eating animal flesh that contains the worm eggs or even the worms themselves
  - Schistosomiasis: liver disease: liver swelling or malfunction accompanied by eosinophilia

▶ Genitourinary system
  » The most obvious defensive mechanism in the urinary tract is the flushing action of the urine flowing out of the system. The flow of urine also encourages the desquamation (shedding) of the epithelial cells lining the urinary tract
  - Urinary tract infections (UTIs): when urine flow is reduced, or bacteria are accidentally introduced into the bladder, infection of that organ (known as cystitis) can occur
  - Discharge diseases with major manifestation in the genitourinary tract: discharge diseases are those in which the infectious agent causes an increase in fluid discharge in the male and female reproductive tracts. Example: *Chlamydia* infection and gonorrhea

- Vaginitis and vaginosis: yeast infection. Inflammation of the vagina
- Prostatitis: an inflammation of the prostate gland
- Genital ulcer diseases: common infectious conditions can result in lesions (ulcers) on the genitals: syphilis, chancroid, and genital herpes
- Wart diseases: The more serious disease is caused by the human papillomavirus (HPV); the other condition, called molluscum contagiosum, has no serious effects
- Group B *Streptococcus* "colonization"—neonatal disease: 10% to 40% of women in the United States are colonized, asymptomatically, by a beta-hemolytic *Streptococcus* in Lancefield group B. Nonpregnant women experience no ill effects from this colonization

Chapter Review Questions

1. The _____ is the time that lapses between an encounter with a pathogen and the first symptoms.
   A. prodrome
   B. period of invasion
   C. period of convalescence
   D. period of incubation

2. Microbiology is
   A. an area of biology that examines dead things that are too small for the naked eye to see.
   B. a specialized area of biology that deals with living things ordinarily too small to be seen without magnification.
   C. a specialized area of biology that deals with living things too big to be seen without magnification.
   D. the study of organisms that live on inanimate objects.

3. Which of the following is *not* a portal of entry for infections?
   A. Skin
   B. Gastrointestinal tract
   C. Respiratory tract
   D. Cardiovascular system

4. Through what process(es) do microbes gain a more stable foothold on host tissues?
   A. Surviving host defenses
   B. Attaching to the host
   C. Adhesion
   D. Both B and C

5. A short period early in a disease that may manifest with general malaise and achiness is called the
   A. period of incubation.
   B. prodrome.
   C. sequel.
   D. period of invasion.

6. Which of the following is a common acquired health care–associated infection?
   A. Surgical site infection
   B. Urinary tract infection
   C. Respiratory tract infection
   D. All of the above

7. Virulence factors include
   A. toxins.
   B. enzymes.
   C. capsules.
   D. A and B.
   E. A, B, and C.

8. What is a symptom of inflammation?
   A. Edema
   B. Accumulation of fluid in an afflicted tissue
   C. Pain
   D. Swollen lymph nodes

9. **What is it called when urine flow is reduced, or bacteria is accidentally introduced to the bladder?**
   A. Vaginitis
   B. Chlamydia
   C. UTI
   D. Prostatitis

10. **What arc dental caries?**
    A. Tooth and gum infections
    B. Tooth decay
    C. Mumps
    D. Periodontal disease

Answers

1. **D.** The period of incubation is the time that lapses between an encounter with a pathogen and the first symptoms.
2. **B.** Microbiology is a specialized area of biology that deals with living things ordinarily too small to be seen without magnification.
3. **D.** The cardiovascular system is not a portal of entry for infections.
4. **D.** Attaching to the host. Adhesion is the process by which microbes gain a more stable foothold on host tissues.
5. **B.** Prodrome is a short period early in a disease that may manifest with general malaise and achiness.
6. **D.** Surgical site infection, urinary tract infection, and respiratory tract infection are all common acquired health care–associated infections.
7. **E.** Virulence factors include toxins, enzymes, and capsules.
8. **C.** A symptom of inflammation is pain. The other choices are signs of inflammation.
9. **C.** Urinary tract infection.
10. **B.** Tooth decay; involves the dissolution of solid tooth surface due to the metabolic action of bacteria.

Reference

Cowan MK, Bunn J, Atlas RM, Smith H. *Microbiology Fundamentals: A Clinical Approach.* 2nd ed. New York: McGraw-Hill; 2016.

4

Surgical Pharmacology and Anesthesia

As an integral member of the patient care team, it is of the utmost importance for the surgical technologist to be familiar with the medications that are administered during the surgical procedure. Additionally, the surgical technologist must be knowledgeable about the indications, contraindications, and safe handling of these medications.

COMMON TERMS

► Agonist: a drug that increases the potency of other drugs
► Antagonist: opposing the action of another
► Indications: the correct treatment or use
► Contraindications: any condition or circumstance that makes a treatment or procedure inadvisable
► Side effect: unintended problems that occur from medications or treatments
► Adverse effect: any unwanted, harmful side effect of a drug
► Toxic effect: the extent to which medications become poisonous to the body
► Tolerance: the act of becoming less responsive to a substance through exposure to it
► Addiction: physical and psychological dependence on a specific substance or practice
► Anaphylaxis: an immediate potentially dangerous allergic reaction, may be severe
► Generic drug names: a drug that is labeled by its chemical name and is not sold under the ownership restrictions of a trade name drug

THERAPEUTIC USES OF MEDICATIONS

► Diagnosis
► Prevention of disease
► Treatment of disease and symptoms
► Anesthetic agents: a drug or chemical that causes partial or total loss of bodily sensation, with or without loss of consciousness

DRUG FORMS

► Gases: oxygen or nitrous oxide
► Liquids: a solution or suspension
► Semisolids: creams, lotions, ointments, suppositories
► Solids: tablets

DRUG SOURCES

► Animals: e.g., heparin sodium (bovine or porcine)
► Minerals: e.g., calcium or iron

▶ Plants: e.g., digitalis
▶ Synthetics: manufactured from laboratory chemicals

ROUTES OF ADMINISTRATION

▶ Enteral
  » Oral: by mouth, placed in the mouth and swallowed (PO)
  » Rectal: placed into the rectum
▶ Parenteral
  » Intra-articular: into the joint
  » Intracardiac: into the heart
  » Intradermal: between the layers of the skin
  » Intramuscular: within a muscle (IM)
  » Intrathecal: into the subarachnoid space
  » Intravenous: into a vein (IV)
  » Subcutaneous: into the adipose tissue layer under the skin (SC)
▶ Topical
  » Buccal: applied to or left to dissolve inside of the cheek (analgesia agents)
  » Dermal: applied to the surface of the skin (topical xylocaine or cocaine)
  » Inhalation: a medicinal preparation administered by inhaling (anesthetic agent)
  » Instillation: a medicinal preparation administered by a catheter or pouring into a body cavity (antibiotic or chemotherapy agent)
  » Sublingual: medication administered under the tongue (digitalis)

COMMON WEIGHTS AND MEASURES

▶ Gram is used for weight or mass
  » 1 gram =1000 milligrams
  » 1 kilogram = 1000 grams
  » 1 kilogram = 2.2 pounds
  » 1 ounce = 30 grams
▶ Liter is for capacity or volume. Commonly used for fluids and fluid measurement
  » 1 liter = 1000 milliliters
  » 1000 liters = 1 kiloliter
  » 1 liter = 1.06 quarts
  » 1 liter = 1000 cubic centimeters or milliliters
  » 1 fluid ounce = 30 milliliters
  » 1 gallon = 3.8 liters
▶ Meter is used to measure length
  » 1 meter = 1000 millimeters = 1.094 yards
  » 1 yard = 3 feet = 36 inches
  » 1 inch = 2.54 centimeters
  » 1 micron = 0.001 millimeter
▶ Abbreviations of weight and measures
  » Centimeter = cm
  » Cubic centimeter = cc
  » Gram = g
  » Kilogram = kg
  » Liter = L
  » Meter = M
  » Milligram = mg
  » Milliliter = mL
  » Millimeter = mm

PREOPERATIVE MEDICATIONS

Opioids are used as preoperative medications and as intraoperative adjunctive agents in balanced anesthesia protocols. High-dose intravenous opioids (e.g., morphine, fentanyl) are often the major component of anesthesia for cardiac surgery.

ANESTHESIA

Anesthesia was first described as "a defect of sensation." In surgery, anesthesia is defined as the total or partial loss of sensation or awareness. The purpose is to incorporate amnesia, analgesia, and pain management to allow for painless surgery.

The type of anesthesia is determined by the anesthetic plan.

Factors include:

▶ Preoperative patient assessment
▶ Proposed anesthesia plan
▶ American Society of Anesthesiologists (ASA) Classification to define risk factors
▶ Elements of the preoperative patient history with emphasis on
  » Cardiac and pulmonary function
  » Endocrine and metabolic issues
  » Coagulation
  » Gastrointestinal
  » Airway management
▶ Other considerations include
  » Comorbidities
  » Age
  » Weight
  » Activity level
  » Medications
  » Allergies
  » Psychological state
  » Emotional well-being
▶ Procedural considerations include:
  » Type of surgery
  » Duration
  » Patient positioning
  » Equipment
  » Surgical site access
  » Surgeon and anesthesia provider preference
  » Patient request

ANESTHESIA TERMS

▶ Analgesia: a state of decreased awareness of pain, sometimes with amnesia. Also defined as the absence of pain
▶ Balanced anesthesia: anesthesia produced by a mixture of drugs, often including both inhaled and intravenous agents
▶ Conscious sedation: technique that combines intravenous agents with local anesthetics, usually used for minor procedures
▶ General anesthesia: a state of unconsciousness, analgesia, and amnesia, with skeletal muscle relaxation and loss of reflexes
▶ Inhalation anesthesia: anesthesia induced by inhalation of drugs

TYPES OF ANESTHESIA

▶ General anesthesia: state of unconsciousness, analgesia and amnesia with skeletal muscle relaxation and loss of reflexes

General anesthesia can be divided into three phases:

1. Induction: begins with induction agents and airway management; intubation (endotracheal tube) or laryngeal mask
2. Airway maintenance: from airway insertion until the completion of the surgical procedure
3. Emergence: at the conclusion of the procedure, anesthesia agents are discontinued; extubation occurs once the patient is breathing on his or her own.

General anesthesia is also categorized into stages.

▶ Stage 1—Analgesia: the patient experiences a decreased awareness of pain, sometimes with amnesia. Consciousness may be impaired but is not lost
▶ Stage 2—Disinhibition: the patient appears to be delirious and excited. Amnesia occurs, reflexes are enhanced, and respiration is typically irregular; retching and incontinence may occur
▶ Stage 3—Surgical anesthesia: the patient is unconscious and has no pain reflexes; respiration is very regular, and blood pressure is maintained
▶ Stage 4—Medullary depression: severe respiratory and cardiovascular depression develops, requiring mechanical and pharmacologic support

ANESTHESIA AGENTS

Inhalation Agents

The agents currently used in inhalation anesthesia are nitrous oxide (a gas) and several easily vaporized liquid halogenated hydrocarbons, including halothane, desflurane, enflurane, isoflurane, sevoflurane, and methoxyflurane. They are administered as gases.

▶ Desflurane: causes vasodilation and decrease in respiratory function
▶ Enflurane: decreases cardiac output and respiratory function
▶ Halothane: decreases cardiac output and respiratory function, increases cerebral blood flow
▶ Isoflurane: causes vasodilation and decrease respiratory function
▶ Nitrous oxide: increase in cerebral blood flow, less likely to cause peripheral vasodilation, decrease in respiratory function
▶ Sevoflurane: causes vasodilation and decrease in respiratory function

Intravenous Anesthetics

When it is difficult to start an IV line in pediatric patients, inhalation anesthetics, such as halothane and sevoflurane, are useful in the induction of anesthesia. Regardless of the patient's age, anesthesia is often maintained with inhalation agents.

Intravenous agents are used in conjunction with inhalation agents or alone depending on the type of procedure or sedation required. These intravenous agents produce hypnosis and include barbiturates, benzodiazepines, etomidate, ketamine, and propofol.

▶ Propofol: produces anesthesia rapidly, and recovery is more rapid than with barbiturates. Possesses antiemetic actions. May cause hypotension upon induction. Causes vasodilation and hypotension
▶ Ketamine: produces a state of dissociative anesthesia. Patient experiences analgesia, amnesia, and catatonia, but consciousness is retained. A cardiovascular stimulant
▶ Barbiturates: (thiopental). Respiratory and circulatory depressants, decrease cerebral blood flow and intracranial pressure. Fast onset, short duration
▶ Benzodiazepines: (midazolam). Used in conjunction with inhaled anesthetics and intravenous opioids. Less depressant effect than barbiturates. Slower onset, but longer duration than barbiturates
▶ Opioids: (fentanyl, morphine). Marked analgesia, respiratory depression
▶ Etomidate: minimal effects on cardiovascular and respiratory functions

Spinal Anesthesia (Figure 4.1)

▶ An injection of local anesthesia below L1 in adults and is sometimes referred to as a subarachnoid block
▶ The needle is advanced through the epidural space and penetrates the dura–subarachnoid membranes, as signaled by freely flowing cerebrospinal fluid
▶ Hyperbaric bupivacaine and tetracaine are two of the most commonly used agents for spinal anesthesia. Both are relatively slow in onset (5–10 min) and have a prolonged duration (90–120 min)

Epidural Anesthesia

▶ Widely used for surgical anesthesia, obstetric analgesia, postoperative pain control, and chronic pain management
▶ Can be used as a single shot technique or with a catheter that allows intermittent boluses and/or continuous infusion

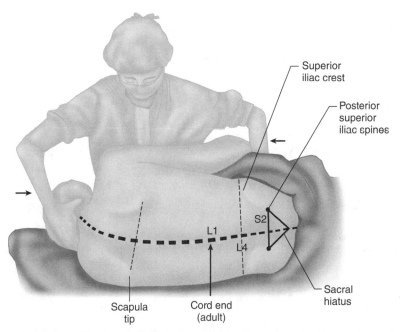

Figure 4.1 Positions and landmarks for spinal anesthesia. (Reproduced, with permission, from Butterworth JF, Mackey DC, Wasnick JD. *Morgan & Mikhail's Clinical Anesthesiology.* 5th ed. New York: McGraw-Hill Education; 2013.)

▶ For the epidural injection the needle passes through the ligamentum flavum and enters the epidural space
▶ Used for surgical anesthesia, obstetric analgesia, postoperative pain control, and chronic pain management
▶ Slower in onset (10–20 min) and may not be as dense as spinal anesthesia
▶ Commonly used short- to intermediate-acting agents for surgical anesthesia include chloroprocaine, lidocaine, and mepivacaine. Longer acting agents include bupivacaine, levobupivacaine, and ropivacaine (Table 4.1)

Regional Anesthesia

▶ Typically injected or applied very close to the intended site of action

Local Anesthesia

▶ Transiently inhibit sensory, motor, or autonomic nerve function, or a combination of these functions, when the drugs are injected or applied near neural tissue

COMPLICATIONS OF ANESTHESIA

General Anesthesia Complications

Aspiration of gastric contents, though rare, is potentially fatal.
Factors for aspiration:

▶ "Full" stomach
▶ Intestinal obstruction
▶ Hiatal hernia, obesity
▶ Pregnancy
▶ Reflux disease
▶ Emergency surgery
▶ Inadequate depth of anesthesia

Interventions to reduce the potential for aspiration perioperatively:

▶ Holding of cricoid pressure (Sellick maneuver)
▶ Rapid sequence induction of anesthesia

TABLE 4.1   Common Local Anesthetic Agents

Agent	Techniques	Concentrations Available	Maximum Dose (mg/kg)	Typical Duration of Nerve Blocks[1]
Esters				
Benzocaine	Topical[2]	20%	NA[3]	NA
Chloroprocaine	Epidural, infiltration, peripheral nerve block, spinal[4]	1%, 2%, 3%	12	Short
Cocaine	Topical	4%, 10%	3	NA
Procaine	Spinal, local infiltration	1%, 2%, 10%	12	Short
Tetracaine (amethocaine)	Spinal, topical (eye)	0.2%, 0.3%, 0.5%, 1%, 2%	3	Long
Amides				
Bupivacaine	Epidural, spinal, infiltration, peripheral nerve block	0.25%, 0.5%, 0.75%	3	Long
Lidocaine (lignocaine)	Epidural, spinal, infiltration, peripheral nerve block, intravenous regional, topical	0.5%, 1%, 1.5%, 2%, 4%, 5%	4.5 7 (with epinephrine)	Medium
Mepivacaine	Epidural, infiltration, peripheral nerve block, spinal	1%, 1.5%, 2%, 3%	4.5 7 (with epinephrine)	Medium
Prilocaine	EMLA (topical), epidural, intravenous regional (outside North America)	0.5%, 2%, 3%, 4%	8	Medium
Ropivacaine	Epidural, spinal, infiltration, peripheral nerve block	0.2%, 0.5%, 0.75%, 1%	3	Long

[1]Wide variation depending on concentration, location, technique, and whether combined with a vasoconstrictor (epinephrine). Generally the shortest duration is with spinal anesthesia and the longest with peripheral nerve blocks.
[2]No longer recommended for topical anesthesia.
[3]NA, not applicable.
[4]Recent literature describes this agent for short-duration spinal anesthesias.

Reversal Agents

▶ Naloxone reverses the agonist activity associated with opioid compounds
▶ Flumazenil is useful in the reversal of benzodiazepine sedation and the treatment of benzodiazepine overdose

Spinal Anesthesia Complications

▶ High neural blockade: spinal anesthesia ascending into the cervical levels causes severe hypotension, bradycardia, and respiratory insufficiency
▶ Cardiac arrest during spinal anesthesia
▶ Spinal or epidural hematoma: symptoms include sharp back and leg pain with a motor weakness and/or sphincter dysfunction
▶ Urinary retention
▶ Backache
▶ Postdural puncture headache
▶ Neurological injury

MALIGNANT HYPERTHERMIA

Malignant hyperthermia (MH) is a rare genetic hypermetabolic muscle disease, occurring 1:15,000 in pediatric patients and 1:40,000 adult patients.

▶ Signs and symptoms most commonly appear with exposure to inhaled general anesthetics or succinylcholine (triggering agents)
▶ Uncontrolled increase in intracellular calcium in skeletal muscle
▶ Sudden release of calcium from sarcoplasmic reticulum removes the inhibition of troponin, resulting in sustained muscle contraction

Early Signs

▶ Tachycardia
▶ Arrhythmias

TABLE 4.2 Protocol for Immediate Treatment of Malignant Hyperthermia

1. Discontinue volatile anesthetic and succinylcholine. Notify the surgeon. Call for help.
2. Mix dantrolene sodium with sterile distilled water and administer 2.5 mg/kg intravenously as soon as possible
3. Administer bicarbonate for metabolic acidosis
4. Institute cooling measures (lavage, cooling blanket, cold intravenous solutions)
5. Treat severe hyperkalemia with dextrose, 25–50 g intravenously, and regular insulin, 10–20 units intravenously (adult dose)
6. Administer antiarrhythmic agents if needed despite correction of hyperkalemia and acidosis
7. Monitor end-tidal CO_2 tension, electrolytes blood gases, creatine kinase, serum myoglobin, core temperature, urinary output, and color, coagulation status
8. If necessary, consult on-call physicians at the 24-hour MHAUS hotline, **1-800-644-9737**

Protocol available at http://www.mhaus.org/nf/Shop/EmergencyTherapyMHPosterSample.png

▶ Hypertension
▶ Mottled cyanosis

Hyperthermia may be a late sign, but when it occurs, core temperature can rise as much as 1°C every 5 min. Generalized muscle rigidity is not consistently present. Hypertension may be rapidly followed by hypotension if cardiac depression occurs. Dark-colored urine reflects myoglobinemia and myoglobinuria.

The drug used in the treatment of malignant hyperthermia is dantrolene sodium, a skeletal muscle relaxant (Table 4.2).

The surgical technologist in the sterile role will assist with patient cooling and Foley catheter insertion. In the nonsterile role, the surgical technologist may assist the surgical team by gathering supplies and assisting in patient transport.

DRUGS ADMINISTERED INTRAOPERATIVELY
Cardiac

▶ Potassium chloride: treatment of or prevention of hypokalemia
▶ Calcium chloride: treatment of hypocalcemia and conditions secondary to hypocalcemia (tetany, seizures, arrhythmias)
▶ Sodium bicarbonate: management of metabolic acidosis, treatment of hyperkalemia. (Improves onset of analgesia and reduces injection site pain when added to lidocaine with epinephrine solution)
▶ Dopamine: increases cardiac output, blood pressure, and urine flow as an adjunct in the treatment of shock or hypotension that persists after adequate fluid volume replacement; in low dosage to increase renal perfusion
▶ Labetalol: for treatment of severe hypertension
▶ Albuterol: treatment or prevention of bronchospasm
▶ Heparin: prophylaxis and treatment of thromboembolic disorders, anticoagulant
▶ Hydralazine: management of severe essential hypertension when oral therapy not possible or when urgent reduction in blood pressure is needed
▶ Papaverine: treatment or prevention of various vascular spasms
▶ Protamine: reverses heparin during surgical procedures

Ocular Medications

▶ Miotics: vasoconstrictor. Used to constrict the pupil and lower intraocular pressure (pilocarpine)
▶ Mydriatics: vasodilator. Used to dilate the pupil (atropine)

Gynecology

▶ Lugol solution: to identify abnormal cervical cells (Schiller test)
▶ Oxytocics: drugs used to contract the uterus either in the induction of labor or follow delivery (oxytocin)
▶ Methergine: causes uterine contraction. Used after delivery, not to facilitate labor

▶ RhoGAM: (Rho(D) immune globulin). Prevention of rhesus (Rh) isoimmunization in an Rh-incompatible pregnancy. Anti-Rh antibody injection given to an Rh-negative woman exposed to Rh-positive blood prevents hemolytic disease of the newborn in a second pregnancy.

▶ Magnesium sulfate: treatment and prevention of hypomagnesemia; prevention and treatment of seizures in severe preeclampsia or eclampsia

DRUG CLASSIFICATIONS/CATEGORIES

Antibiotics

▶ Cefazolin: for **perioperative prophylaxis:** To reduce the incidence of certain postoperative infections in patients undergoing surgical procedures

▶ Gentamicin: treatment of documented or suspected infections caused by susceptible gram-negative bacilli, including *Pseudomonas*, *Escherichia coli*, *Proteus*, *Serratia*, and gram-positive *Staphylococcus*

Intraoperative Solutions, Intravenous Solutions

▶ Dextrose solution 5%, 10%: (5%D, 10%D). Peripheral infusion to provide calorie and fluid replacement

▶ Lactated Ringers (LR): most commonly used intraoperatively intravenous fluid, slightly hypotonic

▶ Normal saline (NS): used for diluting packed red blood cells prior to transfusion.

▶ Five percent dextrose in water (D5W): used as a maintenance fluid for patients on sodium restrictions

Blood Replacements, Substitutes, and Expanders

▶ Albumin: treatment of hypovolemia, plasma volume expansion, and maintenance of cardiac output in treatment of shock and impending shock

▶ Packed red blood cells (PRBC): a centrifuged unit of whole blood, containing approximately 250 mL of packed red blood cells and saline additive (given as a blood transfusion)

▶ Whole blood: contains red blood cells, platelets, and plasma

▶ Dextran: adjunctive treatment of shock or impending shock due to trauma. A priming fluid in pump oxygenators during extracorporeal circulation. (Not a substitution for blood or plasma)

▶ Plasma protein fraction (PPF): plasma volume expansion and maintenance of cardiac output in the treatment of shock or impending shock

▶ Fresh Frozen Plasma (FFP): contains all plasma proteins and most clotting factors used in the correction of coagulopathy

▶ Platelets: transfusion given to patients with thrombocytopenia or dysfunctional platelets in the presence of bleeding

HANDLING OF MEDICATION

Drugs are frequently administered during surgical procedures. They are commonly listed under the surgeon's preferences. Medications are confirmed prior to administration by the surgical team.

The perioperative registered nurse in the circulating role is responsible for obtaining the medication for the surgical patient based on the physician preference card and confirmation with the surgeon.

Prior to administration onto the sterile field, the RN circulator checks the medication:

▶ Label for name
▶ Dose of medication
▶ Prescribed strength
▶ Expiration date
▶ The integrity of the packaging
▶ Color and consistency

The procedure for administration of medication on to the sterile field includes the RN in the circulation role and the surgical technologist in the scrub role both confirming aloud and visualizing:

▶ The medication name on the label of the medication
▶ The dose/strength on medication label
▶ Prescribed dose
▶ Expiration date of medication
▶ The labeled container on the sterile field
▶ A labeled syringe with the prescribed dose/strength of the medication to be administered from the sterile field (for injectable medications)
▶ At the minimum the medication on the sterile field should be labeled with the medication
  » Name
  » Strength/concentration
  » Expiration date
▶ The surgical technologist should place medicine cups and basins close to the edge of the sterile table to avoid the circulator reaching over the table
▶ A distance of 12 to 18 inches should be maintained above the sterile basin to avoid reaching over the sterile field

THE 8 RIGHTS OF MEDICATION SAFETY

1. Right patient
2. Right medication
3. Right dose
4. Right time
5. Right route
6. Right reason
7. Right documentation (including labeling)
8. Right to refuse

Chapter Review Questions

1. Which of the following is an intervention to reduce the potential of aspiration in patients undergoing general anesthesia?
   A. Schiller test
   B. Sellick maneuver
   C. Naloxone
   D. Balanced anesthesia

2. Which of the following drugs is used in the treatment of malignant hyperthermia?
   A. Dopamine
   B. Dextran
   C. Dantrolene
   D. Desflurane

3. Prior to the closure of a CABG surgery, the surgeon says that he would like to reverse the heparin. Which of the following medications will be administered to counteract the heparin?
   A. Protamine
   B. Papaverine
   C. Propofol
   D. Prilocaine

4. This type of anesthesia is often referred to as a "subarachnoid block."
   A. Epidural
   B. Spinal
   C. Local
   D. Balanced anesthesia

5. The early signs of malignant hyperthermia include
   A. tachycardia.
   B. arrhythmia.
   C. hypertension.
   D. mottled cyanosis.
   E. All of the above

6. When added to lidocaine with epinephrine, this solution improves the onset of analgesia and reduces injection site pain.
   A. Sodium bicarbonate
   B. Calcium chloride
   C. Potassium chloride
   D. Dextran

7. Which of the following drugs is a benzodiazepine used in conjunction with inhaled anesthetics and opioids during general anesthesia?
   A. Midazolam
   B. Morphine sulfate
   C. Propofol
   D. Labetalol

8. An example of a common opioid analgesia is
   A. diazepam.
   B. morphine.
   C. propofol.
   D. ketamine.

9. When receiving a medication from the circulator onto the sterile field, the surgical technologist should:
   A. label a container on the sterile back table for the medication.
   B. ask the circulator to read the name of the medication and pour it into a labeled bowl when she/he is ready.
   C. read the name of the drug, strength/concentration, amount of drug, and expiration aloud with the circulator.
   D. have the circulator read the name of the drug, strength/concentration, amount of drug, and expiration to the surgical technologist.

10. Which of the following is the reversal agent for opioid medications?
    A. Flumazenil
    B. Dantrolene
    C. Protamine
    D. Naloxone

11. Cefazolin is given preoperatively to reduce
    A. nausea.
    B. pain.
    C. infection.
    D. aspiration.

12. Which of the following drug is an example of a miotic drug?
    A. Atropine
    B. Pilocarpine
    C. Epinephrine
    D. Lidocaine

13. This drug is thought to be the triggering agent in malignant hyperthermia.
    A. Dantrolene
    B. Succinylcholine
    C. Sevoflurane
    D. Halothane

14. This solution is used to identify abnormal cervical cells.
    A. Sodium bicarbonate
    B. Lugol solution
    C. Magnesium sulfate
    D. Oxytocin

15. Which of the following medications is a treatment and prevention for hypokalemia?
    A. Calcium chloride
    B. Sodium bicarbonate
    C. Magnesium sulfate
    D. Potassium chloride

Answers

1. **B.** The Sellick maneuver is used to reduce the chance of aspiration.
2. **C.** Dantrolene sodium is the medication of choice to treat malignant hyperthermia.
3. **A.** Protamine is the reversal agent for heparin.
4. **B.** Spinal anesthesia is referred to as subarachnoid block.
5. **E.** All are early signs of malignant hyperthermia.
6. **A.** Sodium bicarbonate.
7. **A.** Midazolam.
8. **B.** Morphine.
9. **C.** The circulator and the scrub must perform the steps together and confirm them aloud, acknowledging that both have read all information.
10. **D.** Naloxone is the reversal agent for opioids.
11. **C.** Cefazolin is an antibiotic given prophylactically to reduce surgical site infections.
12. **B.** Pilocarpine.
13. **B.** Succinylcholine.
14. **B.** Lugol solution.
15. **D.** Potassium chloride.

References

Breskin M, Dumith K, Pearsons E, Seeman R. *Medical Dictionary for Allied Health.* New York: McGraw-Hill; 2008.

Butterworth JF, Mackey DC, Wasnick JD. *Morgan & Mikhail's Clinical Anesthesiology.* 5th ed. New York: McGraw-Hill Education; 2013.

Trevor AJ, Katzung BG, Kruidering-Hall M. Opioid analgesics & antagonists. In Trevor AJ, Katzung BG, Kruidering-Hall M, eds. *Katzung & Trevor's Pharmacology: Examination & Board Review.* 11th ed. New York: McGraw-Hill Education; 2016. Available at http://accessmedicine.mhmedical.com/content.aspx?bookid=1568&Sectionid=95702914

Trevor AJ, Katzung BG, Kruidering-Hall M. General anesthetics. In Trevor AJ, Katzung BG, Kruidering-Hall M, eds. *Katzung & Trevor's Pharmacology: Examination & Board Review.* 11th ed. New York: McGraw-Hill Education; 2016. Retrieved February 27, 2016 from http://accessmedicine.mhmedical.com/content.aspx?bookid=1568&Sectionid=95702505.

PART TWO

Patient Care and Safety

5

Medical, Ethical, and Legal Responsibilities

As a member of the surgical team involved in patient care, the surgical technologist (ST) is faced with many challenging ethical decisions. The ST needs to be knowledgeable about medical-legal terms and the ramifications for his or her own actions. The ST needs to be aware of the ethical responsibilities to the patients under his or her care and to consider how decisions and actions may have an impact on the entire surgical team.

LEGAL TERMS

▶ Abandonment: to leave a patient alone who is still in need of care or observation
▶ Aeger primo: "The Patient First" (the motto of the Association of the Surgical Technologists: AST)
▶ Assault: act that causes another person to fear that he or she will be touched in an offensive, insulting, or physically injurious manner without consent or authority to do so
▶ Battery: actual act of harmful or unwarranted contact with a person, including contact without proper consent
▶ Code of ethics: a system of principles intended to govern behavior
▶ Confidentiality: the act of holding information in confidence
▶ Consent: permission from a patient, either expressed or implied, for something to be done by another
▶ Defamation: slander (oral statement) or libel (written statement) that damages a person's reputation or good name
▶ Doctrine of informed consent: the legal basis of informed consent, usually outlined in a state's medical practice act
▶ Doctrine of reasonable man: the principle by which each person is expected to perform his or her job as any reasonable prudent person would in similar circumstances
▶ Ethics: branch of philosophy dealing with good conduct and moral values
▶ False imprisonment: illegal detention of a person without consent (e.g., use of restraints), or forcing a person to stay in an area by not allowing him or her to leave
▶ Intentional infliction of emotional distress: disparaging remarks made about a patient that result in emotional distress
▶ Invasion of privacy: disclosure of private information concerning a patient or photographing a patient without consent
▶ Liable: legally responsible or obligated
▶ Libel: expression through publication in print, writing, pictures or signed statements that injures the reputation of another
▶ Malfeasance: the performance of a totally wrongful or unlawful act
▶ Malpractice: professional misconduct
▶ Negligence: an unintentional tort alleged when one may have performed or failed to perform an act that a reasonable person would not or would have done in similar circumstances

▶ Primum non nocere: "first, do no harm"
▶ Res ipsa loquitur: "the thing speaks for itself," such as a retained surgical item. Also known as the doctrine of common knowledge
▶ Scope of practice: professional duty limits based on state and federal law and on an individual's education and experience
▶ Surgical conscience: the basis for the practice of strict adherence to sterile technique by all surgical team members; involves a level of honesty and moral integrity that must be upheld
▶ Tort: a civil wrong committed against a person or property, excluding breach of contract
▶ Tort law: describes any civil wrong independent of a contract. Tort law provides a remedy in the form of an action for damages. Most actions against operating room personnel are civil actions rather than criminal, for acts that may be either intentional or unintentional

PROFESSIONAL ORGANIZATIONS

▶ Accreditation Review Council on Education in Surgical Technology and Surgical Assisting (ARC/STSA): The mission of ARC/STSA is to provide recognition for the quality of the educational programs in its system to the public. ARC/STSA ensures that programs adhere to accreditation standards with annual reporting of program outcomes.
▶ Association of periOperative Nurses (AORN): A membership-based association providing nursing education, standards, and clinical practice resources—including the peer-reviewed, monthly publication *AORN Journal*—to enable optimal outcomes for patients undergoing operative and other invasive procedures
▶ Association of Surgical Technologists (AST): AST is a membership-based association with the primary purpose of ensuring that surgical technologists have the knowledge and skills to administer patient care of the highest quality
▶ Commission on Accreditation of Allied Health Education Programs (CAAHEP): A postsecondary accrediting agency recognized by the Council for Higher Education Accreditation (CHEA). Carries out its accrediting activities in cooperation with 23 review committees
▶ The Joint Commission (JC): Its accreditation and certification are recognized nationwide as a symbol of quality that reflects an organization's commitment to meeting certain performance standards. Its mission is to continuously improve health care for the public, in collaboration with other stakeholders, by evaluating health care organizations and inspiring them to excel in providing safe and effective care of the highest quality and value
▶ The National Board of Surgical Technology and Surgical Assisting (NBSTSA): Provides professional certification of surgical technologists (CST) and surgical first assistants (CSFA) and promotes quality patient care in the surgical setting

MEDICAL ETHICS

The legal and moral obligations of the surgical technologist are described in the principles of medical ethics. These are the underlying principles of surgical practice and the consent to surgery.

The Four Principles of Medical Ethics	
Beneficence	The obligation of health care providers to help people in need
Nonmaleficence	The duty of health care providers to do no harm
Autonomy	The right of patients to make choices regarding their health care
Justice	The concept of treating everyone in a fair manner

THE SURGICAL CONSENT

▶ Consent: permission from a person, expressed or implied, for something to be done by another
▶ Doctrine of informed consent: the legal basis for informed consent. It is usually outlined in a state's medical practice act

▶ Informed consent implies that the patient understands:
  » Proposed modes of treatment
  » Why the treatment is necessary
  » Risks involved in the proposed treatment
  » Available treatment alternatives
  » Risks of alternative treatments
  » Risks involved if treatment is refused
▶ Items included on the surgical consent:
  » Name of patient, the facility, and surgeon(s) performing the procedure
  » The procedure anticipated to be performed and laterality
  » Permission for photography and/or videotaping or recording of procedure (photographs become part of the medical record)
  » Type of anesthesia
  » Blood products
  » List of complications
▶ Those who cannot give informed consent include:
  » Persons deemed mentally incompetent
  » Persons who speak limited or no English (without the service of an interpreter)
  » Minors
    • Emancipated or married minors may give consent

> Informed consent involves the patient's right to receive all information relative to his or her condition, thus enabling them to make a decision regarding treatment based on that knowledge.

SURGICAL TECHNOLOGIST RESPONSIBILITIES

The surgical technologist participates in three phases of perioperative patient care:

▶ Preoperative: preparation for the patient's care and surgical procedure. This can be in the unsterile role and also in the sterile role with the creation of the sterile field.
▶ Intraoperative: during the surgical procedure at the sterile field
▶ Postoperative: from the time dressings are applied and the procedure is completed. This phase includes management of instruments and equipment and assisting with patient discharge from the OR suite.

SCOPE OF PRACTICE

Core accountabilities of the surgical technologist. Scope of practice for health care professionals is based on:

▶ Education
▶ Experience
▶ National credentialing
▶ State regulations/licensure

TIME OUT: SURGICAL CHECKLIST

▶ All members of the team participate in the "time out" procedure
▶ Initiated prior to the skin incision
▶ Patient is identified upon entrance into the surgical suite, and all team members introduce themselves to the patient
▶ A designated member of the team initiates the procedure after the patient is prepped and draped with the surgical site is visible to all team members
▶ All activity stops for the Time Out procedure
▶ Confirmation of the following is read aloud from the consent:
  » Patient identity
  » Procedure
  » Incisional site
▶ Other items identified:
  » Images
  » Equipment availability/concerns
  » Implant availability

► Anesthesia provider confirms:
- » Physical status
- » Antibiotic prophylaxis
- » Concerns related to medical history, conditions or recovery

► Physician confirms:
- » Anticipated procedure
- » Blood loss
- » Possible changes

► Surgical Technologist and Circulator confirm:
- » Sterilization indicator presence

ETHICAL PRACTICES

The American Hospital Association (www.aha.org) posts the Patient's Bill of Rights at http://www.aha.org/advocacy-issues/communicatingpts/pt-care-partnership.shtml. Here consumers are able to read what a hospital patient can expect in seven languages.

HIPAA

The Health Insurance Portability and Accountability Act (HIPAA) went into effect on April 14, 2003. The standards were developed by the U.S. Department of Health and Human Services (DHHS).

1. Ensure health insurance portability even in the face of preexisting medical conditions.
2. Guarantee the privacy of health information of all patients.
3. Decrease the incidences of fraud and abuse in the health care community.

Key provisions of the standards include:

1. *Access to medical records:* Patients should be able to see and obtain copies of their medical records and request corrections if they identify errors and mistakes.
2. *Notice of privacy practices:* Covered health plans, physicians, and other health care providers must provide a notice to their patients of how they may use personal medical information and their rights under the new privacy regulation.
3. *Limits on use of personal medical information:* The privacy rule sets limits on how health plans and covered providers may use individually identifiable health information.
4. *Prohibition on marketing:* The privacy rule sets new regulations and limits on the use of patient information for marketing purposes.
5. *Confidential communications:* Under the privacy rule, patients can request that their physicians, health plans, and other covered entities take steps to ensure their communications with the patient are confidential.
6. *Complaints:* Consumers may file a formal complaint regarding the privacy practices of a covered health plan or provider.

CONFIDENTIALITY

The surgical technologist must maintain confidentiality of the patient and often colleagues.

► The surgical technologist should only have access to the procedure and patient information for the patients under his or her care
► Patient information should not be discussed with anyone not involved in the care of the patient

ETHICAL CONSIDERATIONS

The surgical technologist may participate in procedures involving moral and ethical concern. Such procedures or situations may include:

► Euthanasia
► End-of-life decisions
► Organ donations and transplants
► Human immunodeficiency virus (HIV)
► Refusal of treatment and palliative care

- ▶ Gender reassignment and transgender patients
- ▶ Abortion and reproductive technology
- ▶ Experimental therapy

SURGICAL CONSCIENCE

- ▶ Rooted in the fundamental understanding of the principles of asepsis and commitment to the application and practice of sterile technique
- ▶ The surgical technologist has a commitment to professional behavior that includes:
  - » Preserving sterile technique
  - » Honesty
  - » Integrity
  - » Patient confidentiality
  - » Nondiscriminatory treatment
  - » Cost consciousness
  - » Providing patient safety

AST CODE OF ETHICS FOR SURGICAL TECHNOLOGISTS

- ▶ To maintain the highest standards of professional conduct and patient care
- ▶ To hold in confidence, with respect to the patient's beliefs, all personal matters
- ▶ To respect and protect the patient's legal and moral rights to quality patient care
- ▶ To not knowingly cause injury or any injustice to those entrusted to our care
- ▶ To work with fellow technologists and other professional health groups to promote harmony and unity for better patient care
- ▶ To always follow the principles of asepsis
- ▶ To maintain a high degree of efficiency through continuing education
- ▶ To maintain and practice surgical technology willingly, with pride and dignity
- ▶ To report any unethical conduct or practice to the proper authority
- ▶ To adhere to the Code of Ethics at all times with all members of the health care team

From the Association of Surgical Technologists. Updated BOD (Board of Directors) January 2013.

Chapter Review Questions

1. Which of the following team members participate in the "Time Out" procedure prior to a surgical procedure?
   A. The surgeon and RN circulator
   B. The surgeon and CRNA
   C. The entire surgical team
   D. The RN circulator and the surgical technologist

2. The surgical technologist in Room 2 thinks that she knows the patient that you just cared for in Room 3. She asks you why the patient needed surgery and what procedure was performed. You tell her,
   A. "I can't tell you any details, but the exploratory laparotomy went well and the patient is stable in the PACU."
   B. "I'm not allowed to tell you, but you can go look at her chart in PACU."
   C. "I can't discuss the patient because you were not assigned, but the exploratory laparotomy for ectopic pregnancy went well."
   D. "I can't discuss any patient information because you were not assigned to the procedure."

3. All of the following can give informed consent except:
   A. Emancipated minor
   B. Person with a diagnosis of Alzheimer disease
   C. Non–English speaking person with interpreter services
   D. A married person 16 years of age

4. Scope of practice is based on all of the following except:
   A. State or federal law
   B. Experience
   C. Education
   D. Professional membership

5. A surgical instrument is left in unintentionally left in a patient. This is an example of
   A. libel.
   B. res ipsa loquitur.
   C. slander.
   D. aeger primo.

6. The four principles of medical ethics are
   A. beneficence, nonmaleficence, justice, and honesty.
   B. maleficence, beneficence, justice, and autonomy.
   C. beneficence, nonmaleficence, justice, and autonomy.
   D. beneficence, nonmaleficence, code of ethics, and autonomy.

7. During the "Time Out" procedure, the surgical technologist and RN circulator confirm
   A. patient's name.
   B. patient's allergies.
   C. surgical procedure to be performed.
   D. antibiotics administered.
   E. All of the above

8. The surgical technologist participates in the preoperative, intraoperative, and postoperative phases of patient care.
   A. True
   B. False

9. **Surgical conscience applies to**
   A. surgical procedures requiring implants.
   B. the first procedure of the day.
   C. all surgical procedures.
   D. only those deemed clean procedures.

10. **Mr. C. signs a consent for a right inguinal herniorrhaphy. Mr. C. receives general anesthesia. While prepping the patient, Dr. Smith notices a mole on Mr. C's right hip. Dr. Smith decides to remove the mole even though removal of the mole is not included on the permit. This would be considered**
    A. improper documentation.
    B. battery.
    C. libel.
    D. res ipsa loquitur.

Answers

1. **C.** All members of the team participate in the "Time Out" procedure.
2. **D.** The surgical technologist should only have access to the procedure and patient information for the patients under his or her care Patient information should not be discussed with anyone not involved in the care of the patient.
3. **B.** Person with a diagnosis of Alzheimer disease.
4. **D.** Membership in a professional organization is voluntary and does not reflect experience or level of education.
5. **B.** Res ipsa loquitur—which means "the thing speaks for itself."
6. **C.** Beneficence, nonmaleficence, justice, and autonomy.
7. **E.** During the "Time Out," at least all of the items noted should be confirmed; the patient's name, patient's allergies, the surgical procedure being performed, and antibiotics administered.
8. **A.** True. The surgical technologist participates in all three phases of patient care.
9. **C.** The surgical conscience applies to all surgical procedures and all patients, every day.
10. **B.** Battery. Since the surgeon did not have Mr. C's consent to remove the mole, this would be considered an act of harmful or unwarranted contact with a person, which in this case was without proper consent.

References

Association of Surgical Technologists. Code of Ethics. www.ast.org

Association of Surgical Technologists. *Surgical Technology for the Surgical Technologist: A Positive Care Approach.* 4th ed. Delmar, NY: Cengage Learning; 2014.

Bodenheimer T, Grumbach K. Medical ethics and rationing of health care. In Bodenheimer T, Grumbach K, eds. *Understanding Health Policy: A Clinical Approach.* 7th ed. New York: McGraw-Hill Education; 2016. Retrieved May 9, 2016, from http://accessmedicine.mhmedical.com/content.aspx?bookid=1790&Sectionid= 121192090.

Hall DE, Angelos P, Dunn GP, Hinshaw DB, Pawlik TM. (2014). Ethics, palliative care, and care at the end of life. In Brunicardi F, Andersen DK, Billiar TR, et al., eds. *Schwartz's Principles of Surgery.* 10th ed. New York: McGraw-Hill Education; 2014. Retrieved June 18, 2016, from http://accessmedicine.mhmedical.com/content.aspx?bookid= 980&Sectionid=59610890.

Judson K, Harrison C. *Law & Ethics for Health Professions.* 7th ed. New York: McGraw-Hill Education; 2015.

6

Infection Control and Aseptic Technique

INFECTION CONTROL TERMINOLOGY

Acquired immunity: formation of antibodies and lymphocytes after exposure to an antigen

Asepsis: exclusion of pathogenic organisms

Bacteriocidal: destroys or kills bacteria

Bacteriostatic: inhibits the growth and reproduction of bacteria

Bioburden: number of microbes or amount of organic debris on an object at any given time

Biofilm: extracellular film produced by an organized community of microbial cells

Community-acquired infection: infection acquired before admission

Cross-contamination: the contamination of a person or object by another

Decontamination: a process to reduce to an irreducible minimum the presence of pathogenic material

Disinfectant: a chemical agent that kills most microbes but not spores on inanimate objects

Event-related sterility: sterility of an item(s) is determined by how a package/container is handled and/or stored rather than time lapse or date. An item is considered sterile until opened or the integrity of the package or container is damaged

Endemic: a disease that is continuously present at subepidemic levels in a particular region, locality, or group. A disease present at fairly low, but constant, level

Epidemic: a disease that rapidly affects many people in a circumscribed period of time, greater than normally occurs in the population

Fomite: an inanimate object that harbors microorganisms

Fungicide: an agent that destroys fungus

Immunity: being resistant to injury and infection by pathogens

Infection: presence of microorganisms in host tissue or the bloodstream

Innate immunity: immunity a person is born with

Nosocomial: infection acquired in hospital

Pandemic: infections that are spread worldwide involving a novel virus and person-to-person spread

Sterile: free of all living microorganisms, including spores (10^{-6})

Sterile field: an area of sterility that is maintained by the surgical team during a surgical procedure

Sterilization: complete killing, or removal, of all living organisms from a particular location or material

Vector: an animate transmitter of disease (e.g., an insect)

FIRST LINE OF DEFENSE

Skin is the first line of defense against infection: a physical barrier (Figure 6.1).

▶ A barrier not easily broken or penetrated
▶ Protects underlying structures
▶ Provides a waterproof barrier
▶ Also key role in body temperature regulation
▶ Mucous membrane: lines body cavities; digestive tract and oral cavity. Also a first line of defense against pathogens
▶ Other defense mechanisms:
  » Cilia in the respiratory system
  » Hairs in the nostrils

SECOND LINE OF DEFENSE (Figure 6.2)

▶ Chemical barriers: lysozymes in tears destroy pathogens that may harm the eye
▶ Inflammatory response:
  » After an incision is made the inflammatory response occurs (Figure 6.3)
▶ Upon incision:
  » Blood vessels in the dermis break and escape into the wound to form a clot
  » Clot consists of the fibrin with platelets, blood cells, and dried tissue fluids
  » Macrophages come into the wound, digest and clean up tissue debris
  » The surface of the clot dries to form a scab, protecting the wound from infection
▶ Five cardinal signs of acute inflammation:
  » Red discoloration
  » Heat
  » Pain
  » Tumor
  » Loss of function

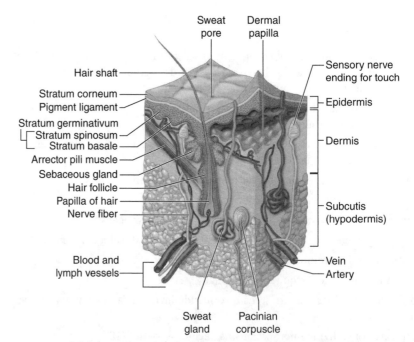

Figure 6.1 Layers of the skin. (Reproduced, with permission, from Brunicardi F, Andersen DK, Billiar TR, et al., eds. *Schwartz's Principles of Surgery*. 10th ed. New York: McGraw-Hill Education; 2014.)

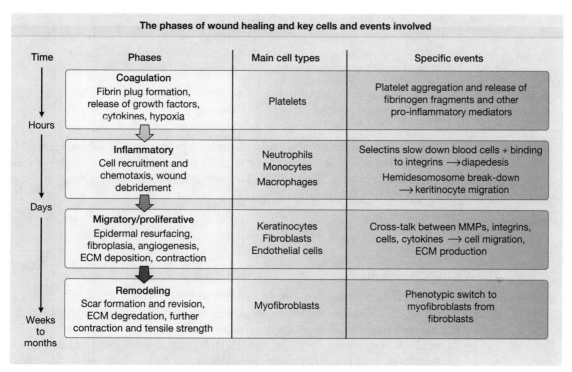

The phases of wound healing and key cells and events involved

Time	Phases	Main cell types	Specific events
Hours	**Coagulation** Fibrin plug formation, release of growth factors, cytokines, hypoxia	Platelets	Platelet aggregation and release of fibrinogen fragments and other pro-inflammatory mediators
Days	**Inflammatory** Cell recruitment and chemotaxis, wound debridement	Neutrophils Monocytes Macrophages	Selectins slow down blood cells + binding to integrins →diapedesis Hemidesomosome break-down → keritinocyte migration
	Migratory/proliferative Epidermal resurfacing, fibroplasia, angiogenesis, ECM deposition, contraction	Keratinocytes Fibroblasts Endothelial cells	Cross-talk between MMPs, integrins, cells, cytokines → cell migration, ECM production
Weeks to months	**Remodeling** Scar formation and revision, ECM degredation, further contraction and tensile strength	Myofibroblasts	Phenotypic switch to myofibroblasts from fibroblasts

Figure 6.2 The phases and events of wound healing. (Reproduced, with permission, from Goldsmith LA, Kats S, Gilchrest B, Paller A, Leffell D, Wolff K, eds. *Fitzpatrick's Dermatology in General Medicine.* 8th ed. New York: McGraw-Hill Education; 2012.)

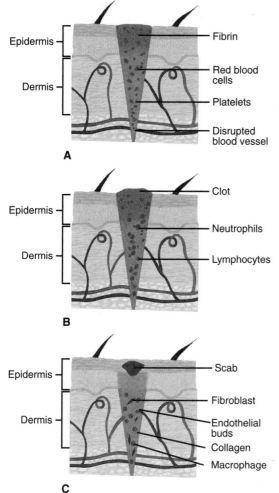

A

B

C

Figure 6.3 The phases of wound healing viewed histologically. **A.** The hemostatic/inflammatory phase. **B.** Latter inflammatory phases reflecting infiltration by mononuclear cells and lymphocytes. **C.** The proliferative phase, with associated angiogenesis and collagen synthesis. (Reproduced, with permission, from Brunicardi F, Andersen DK, Billiar TR, et al., eds. *Schwartz's Principles of Surgery.* 10th ed. New York: McGraw-Hill Education; 2014.)

▶ Causes of acute inflammation:
  » Infection
  » Trauma
  » Physical and chemical agents
  » Necrosis
  » Foreign bodies
  » Immune reactions

The Centers for Disease Control and Prevention (CDC) defines surgical site infection (SSI) as an infection that occurs at or near the surgical incision within 30 postoperative days of the surgical procedure, or within 1 year if an implant is left in place (e.g., mesh, heart valve [www.cdc.gov]). The CDC further classifies SSI as

1. Superficial incisional
2. Deep incisional
3. Organ/space SSI

Wound Classification

▶ Clean wounds: procedures performed for nontraumatic indications, without operative site inflammation, and that do not involve the respiratory, alimentary, or genitourinary tract
  » *Examples: total knee arthroplasty, inguinal herniorrhaphy*
▶ Clean contaminated wounds: procedures in which the respiratory, gastrointestinal, genital, or urinary tract is entered under controlled conditions, without unusual bacterial contamination
  » *Examples: laparoscopic cholecystectomy without bile spillage, abdominal hysterectomy*
▶ Contaminated wounds: procedures with a major break in sterile technique or gross GI spillage, or incisions in which acute, nonpurulent inflammation is encountered
  » *Examples: laparoscopic cholecystectomy with bile spillage, open fracture*
▶ Dirty wounds: old traumatic wounds or existing clinical infection or perforated viscera
  » *Example: incision and drainage of abscess, empyema*

Types of Immunity

▶ Cellular (cell-mediated) immunity: direct form of defense based on the actions of lymphocytes to attach foreign and diseased cells and destroy them
▶ Humoral (antibody-mediated) immunity: indirect form of attack that employs antibodies produced by plasma cells developed from B cells. Antibodies bind to an antigen and tag it for destruction

There are four classes of immunity based on the production or acquisition of antibodies:
▶ Natural active immunity: as a result of normal maturation, pregnancy, or an infection
▶ Artificial active acquired: as the result of vaccination or immunization. (A vaccine consists of either killed or attenuated pathogens)
▶ Natural passive immunity: temporary immunity that results from acquiring antibodies from another individual. This occurs for the fetus through the placenta or for the infant through breast milk
▶ Artificial passive immunity: temporary immunity that results from the injection of an immune serum from another individual or an animal. (Examples are tetanus and rabies serum)

PROCESS OF INFECTION

Infection is the presence of a pathogen in or on the body.

Sources of Infection

External sources of bacteria that can cause infection in a susceptible host include:

▶ Soil
▶ Water

▶ Organic matter
▶ Bacteria
▶ Virus
▶ Toxin
▶ Fungus
▶ Protozoa

Transmission of Pathogens

▶ Direct: transmission of infection; respiratory spread of influenza virus
▶ Indirect: transmission for infection involving a vector such as a mosquito; arboviruses (West Nile virus, yellow fever virus, dengue virus)

Pathogen modes of entry and exit:

▶ Food
▶ Water
▶ Respiratory
▶ Aerosol
▶ Gastrointestinal
▶ Break in skin
▶ Via mucosa or blood
▶ Insect or animal bite
▶ Urogenitalia
▶ Anal or sexual routes

A number of factors determine whether one exposed to a disease will contract it. Host factors that decrease resistance or make one susceptible to infection include:

▶ Age (very young or very old)
▶ Heredity
▶ Preexisting condition (hepatitis B or C, human immunodeficiency virus [HIV])
▶ Nutritional status
▶ Chemotherapy
▶ Steroid use

RISK OF SURGICAL SITE INFECTION

Some of the same factors for host susceptibility are also risk factors for surgical site infection. Risk factors for developing an SSI:

▶ Patient factors
  » Malnutrition
  » Preexisting conditions
    • Diabetes mellitus, cardiac conditions, malignancy, peripheral vascular disease, renal disease
  » Immunocompromised/immunosuppressed patients: those on chemotherapy, HIV
  » Geriatric and pediatric patients
  » Obesity
  » Smoking
  » Anemia
  » Recent surgical procedure
  » Chronic *Staphylococcus* carrier
▶ Procedural factors
  » Inadequate skin antisepsis
  » Inadequate antibiotic prophylaxis
  » Improper sterilization or contamination of instruments
  » Prolonged surgical procedure

Staphylococcus aureus is the most common organism associated with surgical site infections.

ANTIBIOTIC PROPHYLAXIS FOR SURGERY

▶ An antibiotic is selected that has activity against organisms commonly found at the site of surgery
▶ The initial dose of the antibiotic should be given within 30 minutes prior to the incision
▶ The antibiotic should be redosed during long operations based on the half-life of the agent to ensure adequate tissue levels (determined by surgeon and anesthesia provider)
▶ The antibiotic should not be continued for more than 24 hours after surgery for routine prophylaxis

Three factors related to the development of SSIs:

▶ The degree of microbial contamination of the wound during surgery
▶ The duration of the procedure
▶ Host factors such as diabetes, malnutrition, obesity, immune suppression, and a number of other underlying disease states

CLOSURE AND TREATMENT OF SURGICAL WOUNDS (Figure 6.4)

▶ Primary intention: incised wounds that are clean and closed by suture
▶ Secondary intention: wounds with bacterial contamination or tissue loss. These wounds are left open to heal by granulation tissue formation and contraction
▶ Tertiary intention (delayed primary closure): sutures are placed but not fully closed, allowing the wound to stay open for a few days, with subsequent closure of sutures

ISOLATION PRECAUTIONS

▶ Standard Precautions: for all patients
 » Wash hands using a disinfectant soap before and after patient care, including before and after using gloves
 » Put on gloves before contact with skin, mucous membranes, body secretions, excretions, or fluids, and blood
 » Wear mask and eye protection during procedures to protect eyes and mucous membranes
 » Wear a gown during procedures and activities that involve body fluids and/or blood

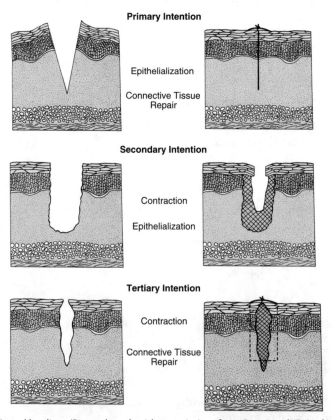

Figure 6.4 Wound healing. (Reproduced, with permission, from Brunicardi F, Andersen DK, Billiar TR, et al., eds. *Schwartz's Principles of Surgery*. 10th ed. New York: McGraw-Hill Education; 2014.)

TRANSMISSION-BASED PRECAUTIONS

▶ Airborne precautions: for airborne diseases (suspected or confirmed TB*, measles, chickenpox):
  » Private negative-pressure patient room
  » Wash hands using a disinfectant soap before and after patient care, including before and after using gloves
  » *Wear N95 mask when entering the patient's room
  » Gloves are worn upon entry into patient room
  » Gown is worn upon entry into patient room
▶ Contact precautions: for infectious diarrhea, wounds infected with *Staphylococcus aureus*
  » Private patient room
  » Wash hands using a disinfectant soap before and after patient care, including before and after using gloves
  » Gloves are worn upon entry into patient room
  » Gown is worn when blood or fluid contact is expected
▶ Droplet precautions: for influenza, pertussis, meningococcal meningitis, and plague
  » Private patient room
  » Wash hands using a disinfectant soap before and after patient care, including before and after using gloves
  » Wear gloves before contact with body fluids or blood
  » Gown is worn when blood or fluid contact is expected
  » Wear mask and eye protection to protect eyes and mucous membranes when within 3 feet of patient

STERILE TECHNIQUE

To prevent or decrease surgical-site infections, sterile technique is employed in the operating room. Sterile technique is the basis of practice for the surgical technologist and the entire perioperative team.

Sterile Conscience

▶ Basis for the practice of strict adherence to sterile technique by the surgical team
▶ A level of honesty and moral integrity is expected that every surgical technologist will uphold in the delivery of patient care
▶ Responsibility to the patient
▶ The ST is responsible for recognizing and correcting breaks in sterile technique when alone or in the presence of others

Aseptic Technique

Surgical attire (OR attire):
▶ Consists of a scrub suit or set of scrubs
▶ Shirt and drawstring tucked in
▶ Close fitting to the body
▶ Changed when visibly soiled or wet
▶ Laundered by approved facility
▶ Scrubs worn outside of the surgical suite are to be changed upon return to the perioperative area

Personal protective equipment (PPE):
▶ Examples include
  » Head coverings
  » Eye protection
  » Masks
  » Shoe covers/impervious boots

Process and system-related factors contributing to higher SSI rates:

▶ Suboptimal choice and timing of perioperative antibiotics
▶ Unrecognized breach of asepsis
▶ Preoperative hair removal
▶ Surgical technique
▶ Operating room traffic
▶ Perioperative hypothermia

---

*American National Standards Institute (ANSI) (2010).

» Nonsterile gloves
» Radiation protection (lead apron)

Sterile surgical attire is:

▶ also considered PPE.
▶ donned after performing the surgical scrub.
▶ includes the sterile gown and gloves.
  » Sterile gown
    • Sterile from the mid-chest to waist
    • Sleeves are sterile circumferentially, 2 inches above the elbow
    • The back is considered unsterile along with the knit cuffs

Traffic Pattern

▶ Unrestricted: non-restricted area—authorized personnel may enter this area in street clothes. Usually the area that leads to the locker room from an outside hospital corridor
▶ Semi-restricted: "Authorized Personnel Only"; OR attire is required in this area. Other PPE includes head covering and shoe covers. Masks may not be required in this area.
▶ Restricted: authorized personnel only in OR attire and PPE, including head covering, shoe covers, and surgical masks. This area usually consists of the surgical scrub sinks, the sterile core area, and individual surgical rooms (operating rooms).

Ventilation

Operating room air-handling systems are laminar air flow system: high-powered unidirectional flow using HEPA filtration to reduce airborne contamination.

▶ Operating room doors should remain closed at all times to maintain the positive pressure in each operating room, creating a higher pressure inside the OR, forcing air out of the room, minimizing airborne contamination
▶ A minimum of 15 air exchanges per hour are required with up to 20 to 25 air exchanges per hour recommended
▶ At least 20% of air exchanges come from outside air

Temperature and Humidity Control

▶ OR temperature is to be kept between 68°F and 73°F
  » Provides comfort for the surgical team and inhibits bacterial growth
▶ Relative humidity range between 20% and 60%
  » Higher humidity can promote mold growth
  » Lower humidity can allow for excessive dust

SURGICAL HAND ANTISEPSIS

▶ Timed or counted stroke method is used when using an antiseptic-impregnated sponge
▶ The brush is not recommended for use on the skin
▶ Timed method requires the hands and arms to be scrubbed for a prescribed length of time
  » Fingers
  » Hands
  » Forearms
▶ Counted stroke method
  » Measured number of strokes are performed for each anatomic area beginning with the fingers and progressing to 2 inches above the elbows
▶ Brushless method
  » Performed in the same order and procedure as other surgical hand antisepsis
  » Follow manufacturer's instructions for use
▶ Waterless method
  » Performed in the same order and procedure as surgical hand antisepsis
  » Follow manufacturer's instruction for use
▶ Surgical hand antisepsis (scrub) procedure
  » Don PPE (surgical mask, protective eyewear, surgical head covering)
  » Remove all jewelry

» Turn on water and wet hands and arms and perform basic hand wash with antiseptic soap, to 2 inches above elbows
» Clean subungual space of each nail under running water and discard nail cleaner
» Rinse hands
» Open surgical sponge, wet and lather
» Begin surgical hand antisepsis at the fingertips. Use the brush and begin scrubbing at the fingertips, incorporating the nails and cuticles. (Brush may be used on fingernail areas)
» Using the sponge, scrub:
   • Each finger, dividing it into four planes and web spaces as a plane
   • The hand, dividing into four planes
   • The arm, dividing it into four planes and three sections and continuing up to 2 inches above the elbow
   • Repeat on the opposite arm
   • Discard the brush
» Begin rinsing with a sweeping motion from the fingertips down the arm keeping fingertips elevated, repeat on opposite arm
» Do not lower the arm, keep fingertips of both arms elevated
» Do not touch any surfaces
» Keep arms bent at elbows and elevated above waist level proceed to OR

PRINCIPLES OF STERILE FIELD

▶ The sterile field is a separate, contained area created within the operating room for the surgical procedure, for a specific patient
▶ Items with in the area are monitored by the members of the perioperative team. These members include the both sterile and nonsterile members of the team
▶ The sterile members include the surgeon, surgical technologist in the scrub role, and the surgical assistant
▶ The nonsterile members include the circulating perioperative nurse, the anesthesia care provider, anesthesiologist, and operating room assistant
▶ Items with in the sterile field are draped and considered sterile. These items are monitored at all times. Items of the sterile field include:
   » Sterile draped back table and all items; instruments, sutures, drapes
   » Draped hand basin
   » Draped Mayo stand
   » Draped patient
   » Draped surgical equipment; microscope, fluoroscope
   » Gowned and gloved surgical team members

Governing Principles

▶ The sterile field is created as close as possible to the time of surgery as possible
   » All sterile fields are monitored at all times and never left unattended
▶ All chemical indicators are examined by the surgical technologist prior to accepting an item to the sterile field
   » Chemical indictors provide assurance that items have been exposed to the sterilization process
▶ Sterile items opened in an OR cannot be move to another OR due to the risk of contamination
▶ The top of the draped sterile procedure table is the only portion that is sterile and can be touched by the sterile ST

DRAPING

▶ Once placed, surgical drapes should not be moved or readjusted
   » Repositioning or moving sterile drapes exposes the sterile field to contamination by raising a contaminated portion of the drape onto the sterile field
▶ Only nonperforating instruments should be used to affix cords or tubing to surgical drapes

» Perforating clamps penetrate the drapes to unsterile areas and create holes, compromising the surgical drape

▶ Impervious drapes should be used to prevent strike-through contamination of the surgical field

» Permeable drapes should be replaced once penetrated by liquid

STERILE AREAS

Scrubbed person:

▶ A separate area is used for gowning and gloving to prevent contamination of the sterile back table

▶ When opening the gown, the 1-inch perimeter of the inner paper wrapper is considered contaminated, and sterile gloves must not be within the 1-inch border

▶ The stockinette of the sterile gown is considered nonsterile and should be covered by the sterile glove cuff at all times

▶ The surgical gown is considered sterile 2 inches in the front below the neckline to table level, and from sterile gloved hands to 2 inches above the elbow

» The back of the gown and any area not visible is considered unsterile

» Changing levels during the surgical procedure alters the sterile gown level

▶ Hands must not fall below the waist or table level

▶ Arms should not be folded with hands in axillary region as this is not a visible area and considered unsterile

▶ Sterile surgical team members pass one another face to face or back to back

» Sterile team members turn their backs to nonsterile areas or individuals when moving around the sterile field

» Movement around the sterile field is kept to a minimum to prevent disruption of airborne contaminants or dust particles

» Talking at the surgical field is kept to a minimum to prevent airborne contamination

▶ Other considerations

▶ Sterile items must remain with sterile items

» Examples include on the sterile field and also supplies in storage areas to prevent confusion or contamination

▶ Nonsterile members must maintain 12 inches from any sterile item including draped equipment

▶ If the sterility of an item comes into question, it should be considered nonsterile or contaminated and should not be used or removed from the sterile field

Chapter Review Questions

1. A laparoscopic cholecystectomy without bile spillage is an example of which type of wound classification?
   A. Contaminated
   B. Clean
   C. Clean contaminated
   D. Clean with reservation

2. The most common organism associated with surgical site infections is
   A. *Geobacillus stearothermophilus.*
   B. *Staphylococcus aureus.*
   C. *Bacillus subtilis.*
   D. MRSA.

3. In the perioperative area, personal protective equipment (PPE) includes
   A. head covering.
   B. eye protection.
   C. mask.
   D. shoe covers.
   E. All of the above

4. All of the following are true about sterile surgical gowns except:
   A. Sterile from the mid-chest to waist
   B. The sleeves are sterile circumferentially 2 inches above the elbow
   C. The back is considered sterile as long as it is visible
   D. The knit cuffs are considered unsterile once the hand passes through and must remained gloved at all times

5. Which of the following statements is true regarding OR ventilation?
   A. The OR doors should remain closed at all times to maintain negative pressure
   B. The OR doors can remain open so that the positive pressure is restored
   C. The OR doors should remain closed at all times to maintain positive pressure
   D. The normal opening and closing of the OR doors will help maintain the negative pressure

6. Before opening supplies in OR 1, ST Bob notices that the room temperature is 69°F and the humidity reading is 45%.
   A. Bob notifies the charge nurse, as the room is too warm and the humidity is excessive. The supplies are in danger due to the high heat and humidity.
   B. Bob records the temperature and notifies the circulating RN.
   C. Bob notes the readings and continues to open supplies, as the temperature and humidity are within normal range.
   D. Bob waits to see if the temperature and humidity will rise before opening supplies, as both humidity and temperature are low.

7. Nonsterile steam members must maintain _____ from any sterile item or draped sterile equipment.
   A. 24 inches
   B. 12 inches
   C. 36 inches
   D. 18 inches

8. Chemical indicators provide assurance that items
   A. are sterile.
   B. have been exposed to the sterilization process.
   C. are aseptic.
   D. are free of bioburden.

9. Which of the following statements is correct?
   A. Repositioning a sterile drape is acceptable prior to securing the bovie or suction.
   B. Perforating towel clips can be used on surgical drapes as long as they are not repositioned or moved during the surgical procedure.
   C. Impervious drapes should be used to prevent strike-through.
   D. When opening the sterile gown, the 1-inch perimeter of the inner wrapper is considered sterile.

10. The top of the draped sterile procedure table is the only portion that is sterile and can be touched by the sterile ST.
    A. True
    B. False

Answers

1. **C.** Clean contaminated.
2. **B.** *Staphylococcus aureus.*
3. **E.** All of the items are considered PPE.
4. **C.** The back of the gown is not considered sterile as it is not visible.
5. **C.** The OR doors should remain closed at all times to maintain the positive pressure.
6. **C.** The acceptable temperature for the OR is 68°F to 73°F and the relative humidity level is 20% to 60%.
7. **B.** 12 inches is the recommended length that a non-sterile team member should maintain from sterile items.
8. **B.** Chemical indicators only show that an item has been exposed to the sterilization process; they do not guarantee sterility.
9. **C.** Impervious drapes are used to help prevent strike-through. All the other statements are false.
10. **A.** True. The top of the table that is visible and in the line of sight.

References

Association of Surgical Technologists. *Surgical Technology for the Surgical Technologist: A Positive Care Approach.* 4th ed. Delmar, NY: Cengage Learning; 2014.

Barbul A, Efron DT, Kavalukas SL. Wound healing. In Brunicardi F, Andersen DK, Billiar TR, et al., eds. *Schwartz's Principles of Surgery.* 10th ed. New York: McGraw-Hill Education; 2014. Retrieved July 23, 2016, from http://accessmedicine.mhmedical.com/content.aspx?bookid=980&Sectionid=59610850.

Beilman GJ, Dunn DL. Surgical infections. In Brunicardi F, Andersen DK, Billiar TR, et al., eds. *Schwartz's Principles of Surgery.* 10th ed. New York: McGraw-Hill Education; 2014. Retrieved July 07, 2016, from http://accessmedicine.mhmedical.com/content.aspx?bookid=980&Sectionid=59610847

Brunicardi F, Andersen DK, Billiar TR, et al., eds. *Schwartz's Principles of Surgery.* 10th ed. New York: McGraw-Hill Education; 2014.

Goldsmith LA et al, eds. *Fitzpatrick's Dermatology in General Medicine.* 8th ed. New York: McGraw-Hill Education; 2012.

Goodman T, Spry C. Prevention of retained surgical items. In *Essentials of Perioperative Nursing.* 6th ed. Burlington, MA: Jones & Bartlett Publisher; 2017.

Kemp WL, Burns DK, Brown TG. (2008). Inflammation and repair. In Kemp WL, Burns DK, Brown TG, eds. *Pathology: The Big Picture.* New York: McGraw-Hill Education; 2008. Retrieved July 23, 2016, from http://accessmedicine.mhmedical.com/content.aspx?bookid=499&Sectionid=41568285.

Rahn DD, McCord E. (2016). Gynecologic infection. In Hoffman BL, Schorge JO, Bradshaw KD, Halvorson LM, Schaffer JI, Corton MM, eds. *Williams Gynecology.* 3rd ed. New York: McGraw-Hill; 2016. Retrieved June 12, 2016, from http://accessmedicine.mhmedical.com/content.aspx?bookid=1758&Sectionid=118166960.

Ryan KJ, Ray CG, Ahmad N, et al. Sterilization, disinfection, and infection control. In Sherris Medical Microbiology. 6th ed. New York: McGraw-Hill Education; 2014. Retrieved June 12, 2016, from http://accessmedicine.mhmedical.com/content.aspx?bookid=1020&Sectionid=56968644.

7

Sterilization and Disinfection

Sterilization and disinfection are concepts that are essential to surgery. These principles are among the basics for the delivery of safe patient care. As with most surgical concepts, it is imperative that the surgical technologist, like all perioperative team members, be knowledgeable about sterilization and disinfection principles.

STERILIZATION AND DISINFECTION TERMINOLOGY

Biological monitors/indicators: a sterilization monitor consisting of a known population of spores resistant to measurable and controlled parameters of a particular sterilization process

Bowie Dick test: a test performed daily to determine whether air is effectively being eliminated from the chamber of a pre-vacuum autoclave. Detects air leaks, insufficient air removal, and steam penetration.

Chemical indicator: an internal or external monitor that changes color when exposed to the sterilization process. Presence of a color change does not indicate sterility of an item, only that the item has been exposed to the sterilization process. Indicators are supplied as a paper strip, tape, label, or marking on an instrument filter.

Decontamination: describes a process that eliminates many or all pathogenic microorganisms, except bacterial spores, or inanimate objects.

Event-related sterility: an item's sterility is determined by the integrity of the package and handling. An item is considered sterile until opened, unless the integrity of the packaging material is compromised.

Immediate-use steam sterilization (previously known as "flash sterilization"): rapid sterilization process of unwrapped items. Done under urgent or emergent circumstances, not to be performed for lack of inventory. Can be performed using prevacuum or gravity steam sterilizers.

Sterilization: removal of all living organisms from a particular location or material. It can be accomplished by incineration, nondestructive heat treatment, certain gases, exposure to ionizing radiation, some liquid chemicals, or filtration.

Ultrasonic cleaning: removes soil by cavitation. Waves of acoustic energy are circulated in solutions to disrupt the particulate matter on surfaces.

Washer decontaminator/disinfector: uses a combination of water circulation and detergent to remove soil. These units provide cleaning, disinfecting, and drying that allow for safe handling of instruments for packaging prior to the sterilization process.

Washer sterilizers: a modified steam sterilizer that cleans by filling the chamber with water and detergent. Steam provides agitation. Instruments are rinsed and experience a short steam sterilization cycle allowing for safe handling of instruments.

DISINFECTION

Chemical Disinfection

▶ Alcohol: Ethyl and isopropyl alcohol are rapidly bactericidal against vegetative forms of bacteria; they are also tuberculocidal, fungicidal, and virucidal, but do not kill bacterial spores. Alcohols are flammable and evaporate rapidly.

▶ Chlorine: Hypochlorites. The liquid sodium hypochlorite is usually called household bleach. It has a broad spectrum of antimicrobial activity. Widely used in healthcare facilities for disinfecting and spot cleaning.

Factors that influence the efficacy of both the disinfection and sterilization process include:

▶ Prior cleaning of the object
▶ Organic and inorganic matter present (bioburden)
▶ Type and level of microbial contamination
▶ Concentration of and exposure time to the germicide
▶ Physical nature of the object (lumens)
▶ Presence of biofilms
▶ Temperature and pH of the disinfection process

Items used in health care facilities are categorized into three classification: critical, semicritical, and noncritical items, also known as the Spaulding classification.

▶ Critical items are used for procedures that enter sterile tissue or the vascular system.
  » Examples include surgical instruments, cardiac and urinary catheters, implants, and ultrasound probes used in sterile body cavities.
  » Items are purchased sterile or sterilized with steam if not heat sensitive.
▶ Semicritical items come in contact with mucous membranes or nonintact skin.
  » Examples include respiratory therapy and anesthesia equipment, some endoscopes, laryngoscope blades, esophageal manometry probes, and cystoscopes.
  » Items require minimally high-level disinfection using chemical disinfectants.
▶ Noncritical items are those that come in contact with intact skin, not mucous membranes.
  » Examples include blood pressure cuffs, operating room beds, and computers.

The first step in the sterilization process is the decontamination process. This process begin in the operating room during the surgical procedure as instruments are wiped cleaned of blood and other bioburden.

At the conclusion of the procedure:

▶ Instruments are opened, cleaned of overt blood and bioburden, channels are flushed
▶ Remove fluids, place instruments in covered, sealed containers, with biohazard warning for safe transport to the decontamination area.

Cleaning is the removal of visible soil from the instrumentation, manually or mechanically, using water with detergents or enzymatic products. This process must be performed prior to the high-level disinfection or sterilization process.

Decontamination Area

▶ Instruments are sorted and decontaminated according to manufacturer's instructions:
  » Handwashing—fiberoptic cables and endoscopic lens and camera systems
  » Ultrasonic washer—fine instruments such as cataract instruments
  » Washer decontaminator—for stainless steel instrument: hemostats, Richardson retractors
  » A neutral pH detergent solution is used for optimal soil removal and material compatibility
  » Enzymes may be added to assist with removal of proteins
    • Care must be taken in thorough rinsing
    • Enzymes can deactivate germicides
▶ Once clean, instruments are sent to the preparation and packaging area where they are inspected, assembled into instrument sets, packaged and sterilized.

Sterile Prep Area

The area in the sterile processing department where the instrument sets are assembled and processed is often referred to as the prep and pack area. This area is the clean area of the department.

▶ Packaging materials/systems
  » Woven fabric
  » Nonwoven materials
  » Paper
  » Peel pack (paper and plastic pouches)
  » Rigid containers
▶ Wrapping of packages
  » Sequentially: two wrappers are folded one at a time to create a package within a package
  » Simultaneously: two wrappers at once; The item is folded into two wrappers to create a single package
▶ Rigid container weight should not exceed 25 pounds

STERILIZATION PROCESS

The five factors crucial to the sterilization process:

1. Time—length of time the sterilant remains in contact with the items for sterilization to occur
2. Contact—all surfaces of the item must be in contact with the sterilant
3. Temperature—the proper temperature must be achieved in order to kill all microorganisms and spores
4. Moisture—a specific amount of moisture must be present to aid in the process
5. Pressure—increases the temperature of the steam so all microbes can be destroyed.

There are multiple types of sterilization. The mode of sterilization is determined by the manufacturer of the instrumentation.

Steam Sterilization (Figure 7.1)

Steam sterilization, saturated steam under pressure, is the most commonly used and inexpensive mode of sterilization used in health care. The process is achieved in an autoclave.

The parameters of steam sterilization are:

▶ Steam
▶ Pressure
▶ Temperature
▶ Time

Common temperatures for steam are 250°F (121°C) and 270°F (132°C).

Pre-vacuum Pressure/Dynamic-Air Removal
▶ A vacuum pump removes almost all air from the chamber prior to injection of steam
▶ Evacuation process creates a vacuum within the chamber
▶ When steam enters the chamber, the force of the vacuum causes instant steam contact with all content surfaces
▶ Steam penetrates every surface instantly
▶ Preset pressure of 27 psi
▶ An exposure time of 3–4 minutes at 270°F–275°F follows the pre-vacuum phase
  » Minimum time for wrapped items is 4 minutes @ 270°F (132°C)

Gravity Displacement
▶ Steam replaces the air in the chamber by gravity
▶ Steam enters the top; because air is heavier than steam, air is forced to the bottom and the steam rises to the top, displacing the air. The air is forced out through an outlet.
▶ Less frequently used in major operating rooms

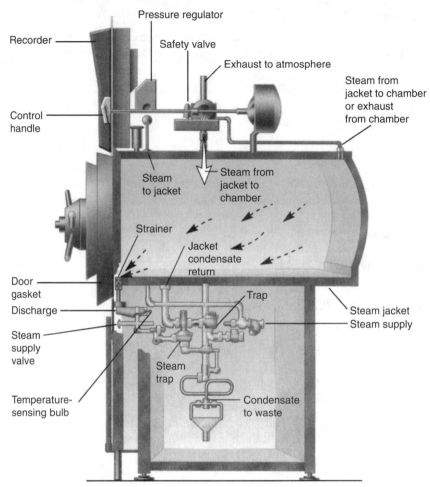

Figure 7.1 Simple form of downward displacement autoclave. (Reproduced, with permission, from Willey JM: *Prescott, Harley, & Klein's Microbiology*. 7th ed. McGraw-Hill, 2008.)

▶ Preset pressure at 15–17 psi
▶ Operated at a temperature of 250°F (121°C) for 15- to 30-minute exposure time for wrapped items

Immediate Use Steam Sterilization (IUSS)
▶ Formerly known as "flash sterilization"
▶ Performed in a rapid manner on unwrapped items needed urgently
▶ Just-in-time sterilization
▶ Performed in specialized IUSS containers
▶ Examples include:
  » 270°F in a pre-vacuum and gravity displacement sterilizer for 3-minute exposure for most metal on non-porous items without lumens
  » Preset pressure of 27 psi
  » 10 minutes at 270°F for items with lumens in a gravity displacement sterilizer
  » 4 minutes at 270°F for items with lumens in a pre-vacuum sterilizer
  » Manufacturer's instructions must always be considered

Ethylene Oxide (EO)
▶ Often referred to as "gas sterilization"; exposes the load to 10% ethylene oxide in carbon dioxide at 50°C to 60°C under controlled conditions of humidity
▶ Exposure times are approximately 4 to 6 hours and must be followed by a prolonged period of aeration (approximately 8 hours) to allow the gas to diffuse out of substances that have absorbed it

▶ Aeration is essential, because absorbed gas can cause damage to tissues or skin
▶ Ethylene oxide is an effective sterilizing agent for heat-labile devices such as artificial heart valves that cannot be treated at the temperature of the autoclave
▶ This method is used less frequently because of the harmful effects of the gas and availability of safer technology
▶ Occupational Safety and Health Administration (OSHA) requires care monitoring of EO cycles and employees in contact. Considered by OSHA as a potential carcinogen, with potential for causing reproductive defects, and irritant to skin and mucous membranes

Plasma Sterilization (Sterrad and Sterrad NX)

▶ In hydrogen peroxide gas plasma sterilization, a plasma state is created by the action of electrical energy on hydrogen peroxide vapor
▶ Used primarily for the sterilization of heat and moisture-sensitive items

Cold Sterilization

Glutaraldehyde (Cidex) is an effective high-level disinfecting agent for apparatus that cannot be heat-treated, such as some lensed instruments and equipment for respiratory therapy:

▶ Commonly used for as a high-level disinfectant for endoscopes and anesthesia equipment
▶ Must be used in a well-ventilated area with daily monitoring
▶ PPE required when handling
▶ Thorough rinsing with sterile water required

Ortho-phthalaldehyde (OPA):

▶ High-level disinfectant sporicidal capabilities
▶ Used on heat sensitive items, endoscopes, transducer probes
▶ PPE required when handling
▶ Thorough rinsing with sterile water required

Peracetic acid (STERIS):

▶ Sporicidal and rapid action
▶ Used in automated machines for endoscopes, dental instruments

MONITORING

Biological monitors: also referred to as spore tests. A method to ensure sterilization.

▶ Steam sterilizers—tested daily using *Geobacillus stearothermophilus* spores
  » Tested in each load containing implants
▶ EO gas sterilizers—tested with each load for *Bacillus subtilis*
▶ Hydrogen peroxide sterilizers—tested daily using *Geobacillus stearothermophilus* spores

Chemical indicators:

▶ Used to monitor one or more process parameters in the sterilization process
▶ A chemical indicator reading of acceptable does not indicate an item is sterile, it means that an item has been exposed to the sterilization process
  » Class 1: process indicator: used in individual packs and containers
  » Class 2: Bowie-Dick test indicator: used for a specific test procedure
  » Class 3: single parameter indicator: used to react to one critical parameter of sterilization
  » Class 4: multi-parameter indicator: used to react to two or more critical parameters of sterilization
  » Class 5: integrating indicator: used to react to all parameters over a specified range of sterilization cycles
  » Class 6: emulating indicator: cycle specific indicator

Physical:

▶ These include monitors on autoclaves such as
  » Graphs or charts
  » Gauges or digital settings
  » Parameter printouts

Other monitors include records of print outs and biological readouts.

DISINFECTANTS

Hydrogen peroxide:

▶ Effective disinfectant for inanimate surfaces.

Iodophors:

▶ Used as antiseptics and disinfectants
▶ Iodine solutions have primarily been used as antiseptics on skin and tissue

Phenolics:

▶ Hospital disinfectant and germicide
▶ Environmental uses, bedside tables, bedrails, and noncritical medical devices

Quaternary ammonium compounds:

▶ Widely used as disinfectants with bactericidal action
▶ Used in environmental sanitation of noncritical surfaces and items that come in contact with intact skin
  » Floors, furniture, and walls
  » Blood pressure cuffs, OR beds

Ultraviolet radiation (UV):

▶ Bactericidal effect
▶ Limited use in the health-care environment for destruction of airborne organisms

Cleaning and Disinfection of Endoscopes

Use of automated endoscope reprocessors (AERs) offers advantages over manual processing as they reduce missed steps in the cleaning process.

▶ Mechanically clean internal and external surfaces, including brushing internal channels and flushing each internal channel with water and a detergent or enzymatic cleaners (leak testing is recommended for endoscopes before immersion).
▶ Immerse endoscope in high-level disinfectant (or chemical sterilant) and perfuse (eliminates air pockets and ensures contact of the germicide with the internal channels) disinfectant into all accessible channels, such as the suction/biopsy channel and air/water channel and expose for time recommended for specific products.
▶ Rinse the endoscope and all channels with sterile water, filtered water (commonly used with AERs), or tap water (i.e., high-quality potable water that meets federal clean water standards at the point of use).
▶ Rinse the insertion tube and inner channels with alcohol, and dry with forced air after disinfection and before storage.
▶ Store the endoscope in a way that prevents recontamination and promotes drying. Hang the scope vertically and a well-ventilated area free of damage and away from high-traffic areas.

Chapter Review Questions

1. Which of the following statements best describes immediate use steam sterilization (IUSS)?
   A. Performed routinely for efficient processing
   B. Done under urgent or emergent circumstances
   C. Used for limited or special equipment
   D. Items can be stored and used for the next procedure if not used on the current procedure

2. The parameters of steam sterilization are
   A. time, temperature, pressure, and speed.
   B. pressure, temperature, time, and solution.
   C. time, temperature, pressure, and steam.
   D. steam, pressure, time, and distance.

3. The most commonly used and inexpensive mode of sterilization in health care is
   A. peracetic acid.
   B. plasma sterilization.
   C. ethylene oxide (EO).
   D. steam sterilization.

4. Steam sterilizers and plasma sterilizers are tested daily using what organism?
   A. MRSA
   B. *Bacillus subtilis*
   C. *Geobacillus stearothermophilus*
   D. *Clostridium tetani*

5. For a pre-vacuum sterilizer the minimum exposure time is 4 minutes with a minimum temperature of _____.
   A. 250°F
   B. 121°F
   C. 132°F
   D. 270°F

6. The ultrasonic washer cleans instrument by which of the following mechanisms?
   A. Agitation
   B. Cavitation
   C. Enzymatic action
   D. Decalcification

7. If a sterile wrapped item falls on the floor, what action should be taken?
   A. Use the item if the wrapper intact
   B. Open the item and send it to Sterile Processing for re-processing
   C. Return the item to the shelf in the storage area
   D. Ask your co-worker to use the item next

8. Which of the following methods is not recommended for sterilizing flexible endoscopes and fiberoptic light cords?
   A. Peracetic acid
   B. Ethylene oxide
   C. Steam
   D. Glutaraldehyde

9. Which of the following tests is performed on pre-vacuum sterilizers to detect air leaks?
   A. Biological monitor test
   B. Bowie-Dick test
   C. Chemical indicator test
   D. Pressure gauge test

10. Which of the following best describes "event-related" sterility?
    A. Consider the item sterile until opened
    B. Consider the item sterile if the item is not outdated
    C. Consider the item sterile until opened, unless the integrity of the packaging material is compromised
    D. Consider the item sterile if sealed and not outdated

11. An example of a critical patient care item is
    A. a laryngoscope.
    B. a Kelly clamp.
    C. a blood pressure cuff.
    D. an operating room bed.

12. An example of a semi-critical patient care item is
    A. a laryngoscope.
    B. a Kelly clamp.
    C. a blood pressure cuff.
    D. an operating room bed.

13. The autoclave tape used on packaging is considered which class of indicator?
    A. Class 1
    B. Class 2
    C. Class 3
    D. Class 4

14. The first step in the sterilization process is
    A. contain.
    B. disassemble.
    C. decontamination.
    D. dispense.

15. The term describing the absence of all microbial life including spores is
    A. aseptic.
    B. sterile.
    C. disinfected.
    D. decontaminated.

Answers

1. **B.** IUSS is only performed under emergent or urgent circumstances. Items cannot be stored; they must be for immediate use.
2. **C.** The parameters for steam sterilization are time, temperature, pressure, and steam.
3. **D.** Steam sterilization is the most commonly used and inexpensive mode of sterilization in health care today. It is readily available and inexpensive to operate.
4. **C.** *Geobacillus stearothermophilus* is the spore used to test the efficiency of the sterilizer.
5. **D.** 270°F.
6. **B.** Cavitation.
7. **B.** If in doubt, the item should not be used. Open the item and send it to Sterile Processing for reprocessing.
8. **C.** Steam is not recommended for use on flexible endoscopes or fiberoptic light cords.
9. **B.** The Bowie-Dick test is used to detect air leaks, insufficient air removal, and steam penetration.
10. **C.** Consider the item sterile until opened, unless the integrity of the packaging material is compromised.
11. **B.** Kelly clamp. Any item that enters a sterile cavity is a critical item.
12. **A.** Laryngoscope. Any item that enters a mucous membrane is a semi-critical item.
13. **A.** Class 1 indicator.
14. **C.** Decontamination is the first step in the sterilization process and begins in the OR.
15. **B.** Sterility is considered the absence of all microbial life including spores.

References

Goodman T, Spry C. Instrument processing. In *Essentials of Perioperative Nursing.* 6th ed. Burlington, MA: Jones & Bartlet Publisher; 2017.

Rutala WA, Weber DJ. Healthcare Infection Control Practices Advisory Committee (HICPAC). Guideline for Disinfection and Sterilization in Healthcare Facilities, 2008. Washington, DC: Centers for Disease Control and Prevention; 2008.

Ryan KJ, Ray C. Sterilization, disinfection, and infection control. In Ryan KJ, Ray C, eds, *Sherris Medical Microbiology.* 6th ed. New York: McGraw-Hill; 2014. Retrieved from http://accessmedicine.mhmedical.com/content.aspx?bookid=1020&Sectionid=56968644

Willey JM. *Prescott, Harley, & Klein's Microbiology.* 7th ed. New York: McGraw-Hill, 2008.

PART THREE

Preoperative Preparation

8

The Surgical Team

The surgical team or perioperative team consists of both sterile and nonsterile team members. An entire team is required to care for one patient throughout the perioperative experience.

PERIOPERATIVE TEAM MEMBERS
Sterile Team Members
▶ Operating surgeon (MD, DO, DPM, DDS)
▶ First assistant to the surgeon (MD or DO), surgical resident, RNFA, CSFA
▶ Scrub person—surgical technologist or RN

Nonsterile Team Members
▶ Circulator—RN
▶ Anesthesia care provider
   » Anesthesiologist (MD or DO), Certified Registered Nurse Anesthetist (CRNA)
▶ Operating Room Assistant (ORA)/Orderly
▶ Perfusionist
▶ Radiology Technologist
▶ Other members not physically present in the OR include:
   » Charge Nurse (coordinating the OR schedule and patient care from the front desk)
   » Pathologist
   » Radiologist

RESPONSIBILITIES OF THE SURGEON
▶ Obtains the surgical consent
   » Discusses the risks and benefits of the procedure
   » Alternative treatment
▶ Marks the surgical site
▶ Confirms the surgical plan with the perioperative team
   » Pre-procedure huddle
▶ Participates in or initiates the surgical "Time Out"
▶ Identifies the surgical site
▶ Performs the surgical procedure
▶ Provides postoperative care

Responsibilities of the Surgical Assistant
▶ Assesses the patient preoperatively
▶ Assists in positioning the patient
▶ Preps the patient

▶ Drapes the patient
▶ Participates in the "Time Out" procedure
▶ Provides visualization through
  » Tissue retraction
  » Suctioning
  » Sponging
▶ Provides hemostasis
▶ Sutures
▶ Identifies surgical anatomy
▶ Places drains
▶ Applies dressings
▶ Assists in patient transport

RESPONSIBILITIES OF THE SURGICAL TECHNOLOGIST IN THE SCRUBBED ROLE

Preoperative Patient Care

▶ Prepares the OR for the surgical patient
  » Gathers supplies and equipment specific for the surgical procedure
  » Opens sterile supplies and instruments
  » Creates a sterile field
  » Performs surgical antisepsis and dons a sterile gown and gloves
  » Prepares the sterile field/back table for the procedure
  » Performs the surgical counts with the circulating RN

Intraoperative Patient Care

▶ Gowns and gloves surgical team members
▶ Actively participates in the "Time Out" procedure
▶ Assists with the draping procedure
▶ Prepares all surgical equipment for the start of the procedures
  » Suction, electrocautery, and Mayo stand
▶ Maintains and monitors the sterile field throughout the procedure
▶ Establishes a neutral zone for sharps
▶ Assesses and anticipates the needs of the patient and surgeon throughout the surgical procedure
  » Passes instruments
  » Prepares instruments in ready
  » Loads suture and stapling devices
  » Prepares medications for safe handling
  » Ensures readiness of irrigation
  » Prepares for surgical counts
  » Counts items added to surgical field
▶ Ensures the safe handling of surgical specimen
▶ Initiates surgical counts
▶ Places sterile dressing

Postoperative Patient Care

▶ Maintains the sterile field until the patient is transported from the OR
▶ Secures sharps and discards them in the proper container
▶ Disassembles instruments and contains them for transport to the decontamination area in approved containers
▶ Assists the perioperative team with room cleaning and preparation for the next patient

RESPONSIBILITIES OF THE RN CIRCULATOR

▶ Prepare the OR for the surgical procedure
▶ Assesses the patient in the preoperative area
▶ Reviews patient chart
  » Confirms surgical consent

- » Verifies patient identification
- » Reviews diagnostic and laboratory results
- ▶ Confirms that all diagnostic and laboratory reports are available
- ▶ Assists with patient transport to OR and transfer to OR bed
- ▶ Verifies patient identification with perioperative team members
- ▶ Assists the anesthesia provider as needed
- ▶ Assists with patient positioning
- ▶ Initiates and/or participates in the "Time Out" procedure as facility procedure indicates
- ▶ Performs the surgical count with the surgical technologist
- ▶ Performs the patient prep
- ▶ Monitors the sterile field and assists all members of the sterile team
- ▶ Completes perioperative patient documentation
- ▶ Secures surgical specimens handed off from the operative field
- ▶ Assists with dressings
- ▶ Assists with the transfer of the patient from the OR bed postprocedure
- ▶ Transports the patient to the postanesthesia care unit (PACU)

RESPONSIBILITIES OF THE ANESTHESIA CARE PROVIDER

- ▶ Preoperative patient assessment
- ▶ Determines the anesthesia plan—the type of anesthesia to be administered specific to the needs of the patient and procedure
- ▶ Obtains informed consent
  - » Discusses anesthesia risks and benefits
- ▶ Manages the patient throughout all phases of anesthesia
  - » Monitors vital signs
  - » Manages airway and fluids
  - » Ensures patient's comfort through pain management

The #1 priority of all perioperative team members in transport is the patient's airway.

RESPONSIBILITIES OF THE SURGICAL TECHNOLOGIST IN THE CIRCULATING ROLE OR ASSISTING THE CIRCULATING

(This role may vary from state to state.) The surgical technologist may be called upon to assist the circulating nurse such as in an emergency situation.

Duties may include:

- ▶ Preparing the room for the surgical procedure
- ▶ Gathering additional supplies and equipment
- ▶ Assisting with transfer of the patient
- ▶ Positioning the patient
- ▶ Opening sterile supplies
- ▶ Taking specimens to the laboratory
- ▶ Facilitating needed services such as radiology
- ▶ Communicating with the charge nurse and other service providers
- ▶ Assisting the anesthesia provider

THE POSTANESTHESIA UNIT (PACU)

The PACU is where the patient is taken to be managed after the surgical procedure. The patient is received by the PACU RN. The most important aspects of patient care in the PACU is monitoring of airway (if applicable) and vital signs. Some patients arrive in the PACU still intubated (with the endotracheal tube in place).

Responsibilities of the PACU RN include

- ▶ Receive report/SBAR from anesthesia provider
- ▶ Patient identification with two health care providers
- ▶ Assessment of patient airway and vital signs
  - » Pulse oximeter to monitor oxygen saturation
  - » Blood pressure cuff-blood pressure
  - » Electrocardiogram monitor (ECG) to monitor heart rate and rhythm
- ▶ Oxygen is usually administered upon arrival in the PACU

- ▶ IV site and fluids are assessed
- ▶ Incision site, drains and catheters are assessed
- ▶ Warm blankets applied
- ▶ pain medication need is assessed
- ▶ Patients are discharge from PACU upon meeting discharge criteria based on the Aldrete Score

SBAR a communication technique for patient hand off

S—Situation
B—Background
A—Assessment
R—Recommendation

TEAM AND PERSONAL QUALITIES AND REQUIREMENTS OF THE SURGICAL TECHNOLOGIST

- ▶ Communicates effectively
- ▶ Is respectful of patients' and team members' rights and privacy
- ▶ Works well with others in a complex environment
- ▶ Possesses stamina and manual dexterity to handle complex instrumentation
- ▶ Able to prioritize
- ▶ Adapts to change
- ▶ Detail oriented
- ▶ Eager to learn
- ▶ Works efficiently and accurately
- ▶ Dependable
- ▶ Able to identify practice issues and take corrective measures quickly
- ▶ Able to establish and maintain effective working relationships with patient care team members in the perioperative setting and beyond
- ▶ Establishes effective communication and rapport with patient and family
- ▶ Functions effectively under stress and in emergency situations

Chapter Review Questions

1. Sterile perioperative team member include all of the following except:
   A. surgeon.
   B. first assistant.
   C. surgical technologist.
   D. CRNA.

2. Intraoperative responsibilities of the surgical technologist in the scrubbed role include:
   A. establishing a neutral sharps zone.
   B. passing instruments.
   C. counting items added to the sterile field.
   D. completing perioperative paper work.

3. The RN circulator responsibilities include all of the following except:
   A. preoperative patient assessment.
   B. obtaining the surgical consent.
   C. assisting with positioning.
   D. initiating and/or participating in the "Time Out" procedure.

4. Positioning for the surgical procedure includes all of the following team members except:
   A. the surgical first assistant.
   B. the anesthesia care provider.
   C. the PACU RN.
   D. the circulating perioperative RN.

5. A communication technique used to relay patient information from one staff member to another is called:
   A. Aldrete.
   B. SBAR.
   C. Time Out.
   D. huddle.

Answers

1. **D.** The CRNA is the anesthesia provider and is an unsterile member of the perioperative team.
2. **D.** The perioperative RN in the circulator role is responsible for the perioperative paperwork.
3. **B.** The surgeon is responsible for obtaining the consent. The RN circulator can witness the consent.
4. **C.** The PACU RN does not assist with the positioning of the patient for the surgical procedure.
5. **B.** SBAR is a communication technique used to communicate information about a patient from one staff member to another.

9

Patient Positioning

CONSIDERATIONS FOR PATIENT POSITIONING

The OR bed:

- ▶ General function
  - » Electric vs. non-electric functioning
  - » Elevation
  - » Locking and unlocking
  - » Kidney rest
  - » Side tilt
  - » Head of bed elevation
  - » Lowering and raising the foot of the bed
- ▶ Accessories
  - » Arm boards and straps
  - » Stirrups
  - » Leg extenders
  - » Foot boards
  - » Side extensions—bariatric considerations
  - » Gel pads
  - » Horseshoe head positioner (prone positioning)
  - » Foam padding
  - » Pillows
  - » Vacuum positioning devices
- ▶ Additional supports and supplies
- ▶ Specialty OR beds are available
  - » Fracture beds
  - » Spinal positioning devices

Factors influencing patient positioning:

- ▶ Type of anesthesia
- ▶ Surgeon preference
- ▶ Patient consideration—limitations
- ▶ Physiological and anatomical considerations
- ▶ Safety
- ▶ Procedure and incision site

POSITIONS

Supine (dorsal recumbent)

- ▶ The most common surgical position
- ▶ Patient is positioned flat on back, head and spine in horizontal alignment

▶ Hips parallel with legs in a straight line uncrossed
▶ Head positioned on a pillow or head read
▶ Arms positioned at side or on arm board not extended past 90° angle to avoid a brachial plexus injury
▶ The safety strap is placed 2 inches above the knees

Variations

▶ Trendelenburg
  » Supine position with the OR bed tilted head down; the patient's feet are higher than the patient's head
  » Used in laparoscopic and open abdominal procedures to visualize organs of the lower abdominal cavity and in patients with hypovolemic shock
▶ Reverse Trendelenburg
  » Supine position with the OR bed tilted feet down; the head is higher than the patient's feet
  » Used for head and neck surgery, open and laparoscopic abdominal procedures to visualize organs of the upper abdominal cavity
▶ Lithotomy
  » Supine position with the legs elevated and abducted in stirrups
  » The buttocks are even with the lower break in the OR bed, allowing for lowering of the foot of the bed. Position of hands must be noted when the foot of bed is lowered to avoid injury
  » Used for procedures of the perineum, pelvic organs, and genitalia
  » Care must be taken when raising and lowering legs into stirrups
    • Two people position legs
    • Legs are brought together and raised and positioned in stirrups
    • At the conclusion, legs are brought together and lowered one at a time to prevent injury and sudden changes in blood pressure
▶ Fowler (semi-Fowler, semi-sitting, beach chair) (Figure 9.1)
  » The modification of sitting position can be used for some craniotomy and shoulder procedures
  » The head is supported along with padded footrest
  » Additional padding is provided to the lower back, ischial tuberosities and under the knees
  » Safety strap is placed 2 inches above the knees

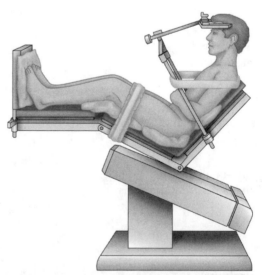

Figure 9.1 Semi-Fowler's, Semi-sitting, or Beach Chair position. (Reproduced, with permission, from Butterworth JF, Mackey DC, Wasnick JD. *Morgan & Mikhail's Clinical Anesthesiology*. 5th ed. New York: McGraw-Hill Education; 2013.)

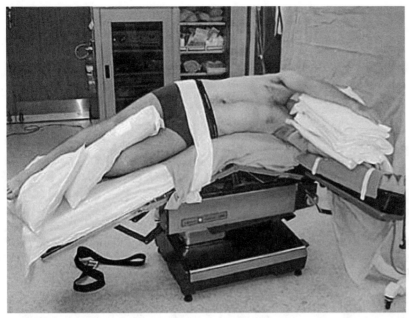

Figure 9.2 Lateral position. (Kidney position). (Reproduced, with permission, from Brunicardi FC et al., eds. *Schwartz's Principles of Surgery*. 10th ed. New York: McGraw-Hill Education; 2015.)

Lateral (lateral decubitus) (Figure 9.2)

▶ Also known as the kidney position: the patient lies on one side
▶ Used for surgery of the kidney, retroperitoneal space, access to the thorax and hip
▶ Right lateral
  » Patient lies on the right side for surgery on the left
▶ Left lateral
  » Patient lies on the left side for surgery on the right
▶ A pillow is placed between the legs
▶ The upper leg is straight and the lower leg is flexed
▶ The head must be in cervical alignment with the spine
▶ Care is taken with the arms; an elevated arm board is used for the upper arm
▶ An axillary roll is placed under the lower axilla
▶ Sims-
  » Used during colonoscopy (left lateral)

Prone

▶ The patient is positioned on the abdomen for procedures involving the spine, back, rectum, and posterior aspects of the extremities
▶ Pillows or rolls may be used in addition to chest rolls
▶ Patients are usually placed under anesthesia on the stretcher and "log rolled" on to the OR bed by a minimum of four perioperative team members
  » The 1st team member (usually the anesthesia provider) supports the head and protects the patient's airway
  » 2nd team member (person on left side of patient) rolls the patient from the stretcher to chest rolls or frame of the arms of
  » 3rd team member (person on right side of patient) supports the patient's chest and lower abdomen
  » 4th team member (person at the foot of patient) supports and turns the patient's legs
▶ Kraske/Jacknife (Figure 9.3)
  » A variation of the prone position with the OR bed flexed at the center break
  » Used for rectal procedures
▶ Knee-chest
  » May be used for lumbar laminectomy or sigmoidoscopy
  » Table is flexed at the center break, with the leg section at right angles; a foot extension is used

Prior to moving a patient always confirm with the anesthesia provider. The airway must be secured and monitored prior to any move. It is a team effort.

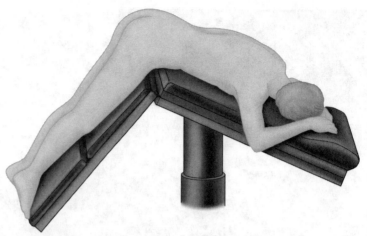

Figure 9.3 Jacknife or Kraske Position. (Reproduced, with permission, from Butterworth JF, Mackey DC, Wasnick JD. *Morgan & Mikhail's Clinical Anesthesiology.* 5th ed. New York: McGraw-Hill Education; 2013.)

SURGICAL SKIN PREP

As the skin serves as the primary barrier to infection, the skin must be prepared prior to the surgical procedure. Surgical antisepsis may begin 24 hours prior to surgery according the surgeon's preference.

► A surgical clip (electric clipper) may also be necessary. Clipping should be performed prior to entering the operating room (as close to surgery as possible). Razors may not be used. Surgical depilatory creams may be used. A skin test is performed for skin sensitivity.

Surgical antiseptic solutions:

► Iodophors and iodine
  » Used as antiseptics and disinfectants
► Chlorhexidine gluconate (CHG)
► Alcohol preparation (60% to 90%)

Considerations include:

► Patient allergy and sensitivity to product
► Area to be prepped
► Manufacturer's recommendations
► Dry time
► Flammability—all products containing alcohol must be allowed to dry a minimum of 3 minutes prior to draping
► Pooling of products—can cause skin irritation and burns to patients

Principles of prepping:

► Ensure that all materials needed are available
► A separate prep table may be used
  » Drape a sterile prep table
  » Sterile gloves
  » Prep cups, sponges and solution or prep sticks (for contained solution systems)
  » Counted sponges required for vaginal preps
  » Sterile towel
► Begin prep at the intended incision site and work toward the periphery, such as in a circular motion on the abdomen
► Umbilicus is cleaned separately with cotton-tip applicators
► Colostomy or stomas are covered
► A separate setup is used for perineal and abdominal prep
  » The abdominal prep is performed first

CHG cannot be used near the eye, ear or on mucous membranes.

If the patient's head is shaved for neurosurgery, the hair must be saved. It is considered one of the patient's belongings.

Chapter Review Questions

1. The minimum number of team members required to safely transfer a patient from a stretcher to the OR bed?
   A. 3
   B. 2
   C. 4
   D. 6

2. The most common surgical position utilized is
   A. Semi-Fowler's
   B. Supine (dorsal recumbent)
   C. Prone
   D. Lithotomy

3. A common surgical position utilized for gynecological or perineum procedures is
   A. Lithotomy
   B. Prone
   C. Supine (dorsal recumbent)
   D. Kraske/Jacknife

4. This position is used for patient's in hypovolemic shock and in laparoscopic procedures to visualize the pelvic organs.
   A. Reverse Trendelenburg
   B. Trendelenburg
   C. Lateral decubitus
   D. Fowler's

5. Principles of skin prepping include all of the following except
   A. Avoid pooling of products
   B. Do not allow product to dry before draping
   C. Check patient allergy
   D. Begin the prep at the incision site and move outward

6. The patient is scheduled for a left nephrectomy, the ST know that patient will be positioned in
   A. Left lateral position
   B. Right lateral position
   C. Jackknife position
   D. Prone position

7. What is the proper placement of the safety strap on the patient positioned on the OR bed in supine position?
   A. Across the abdomen
   B. 2 inches above the knees
   C. Across the pelvis
   D. 2 inches below the knees

8. Which of the following statements is true when positioning a patient in the dorsal recumbent position?
   A. Safety strap is positioned 2 inches below the knees
   B. Hips are parallel and in a straight line and legs are uncrossed
   C. An axillary roll is placed under the lower axilla
   D. Arms are positioned on arm boards at 100°–120° angle

9. During a thyroidectomy what position would be utilized to assist in visualization?
   A. Trendelenburg
   B. Sims
   C. Kraske
   D. Reverse Trendelenburg

10. The next procedure scheduled in your room is a D&C. You know the patient will be in _____ position and you will need _____ to position the patient.
    A. Kraske, gel rolls
    B. Sims, stirrups
    C. Lithotomy, stirrups
    D. Lateral, stirrups

Answers

1. **C.** A minimum of 4 team members are required to move a patient safely, one at the head, one on either side of the patient and one at the foot.

2. **B.** Supine (dorsal recumbent) is the most common surgical position utilized

3. **A.** Lithotomy

4. **B.** Trendelenburg

5. **B.** To avoid surgical fires and patient skin injury, all surgical skin prep solutions should dry completely before draping

6. **B.** Right lateral position. The patient is positioned with the right side down and the operative side, left is up.

7. **B.** The safety strap is placed 2 inches above the knees when the patient is positioned in the supine position.

8. **B.** In dorsal recumbent (supine) position the hips are parallel and in a straight line and legs are uncrossed.

9. **D.** Reverse Trendelenburg allows for the visualization of neck structures with the held elevated and the feet lowered.

10. **C.** The patient will be positioned in Lithotomy position and stirrups are used for D&C procedures.

References

Butterworth JF, Mackey DC, Wasnick JD. *Morgan & Mikhail's Clinical Anesthesiology.* 5th ed. New York: McGraw-Hill Education; 2013.

Brunicardi FC et al., eds. *Schwartz's Principles of Surgery.* 10th ed. New York: McGraw-Hill Education; 2015.

Goodman T, Spry C. Prevention of retained surgical items. In *Essentials of Perioperative Nursing.* 6th ed. Burlington, MA: Jones & Bartlet Publisher; 2017.

10

Surgical Supplies

DRAPES

▶ Drape Materials
  » Nonwoven fabrics: Disposable; typically made from compressed synthetic fibers, such as nylon or polyester bonded with cellulose
    • Disposable drapes have reinforced layers of material surrounding the fenestration (opening) of the drape
    • Some may have a plastic cover with a central slit over a rounded fenestration for snug fits around extremities
  » Woven textile fabrics
    • Reusable drapes are popular with hospitals because they are cheaper to use than disposable drapes
    • The cotton fibers of the material swell when they become wet, making the material impermeable to liquids
    • Reusable drapes have certain disadvantages: must be laundered, folded, inspected for wear, and sterilized after each use
    • Because they are reusable, the handlers' risk of exposure to contaminants is increased
  » Plastic adhesive drapes: made of a thin, clear, plastic material that has an adhesive backing and can be applied to the skin without blocking vision
  » Incise drapes
    • Have an adhesive backing that may be impregnated with an antimicrobial iodine agent that is slowly released after application to destroy bacteria from the patient's skin during the surgical procedure
    • The prepped skin should be allowed to sufficiently dry so that the incise drape sticks properly
  » Aperture drapes
    • Small clear plastic drapes with openings that are surrounded by an adhesive backing
    • Used to drape eyes and ears and allow the surgeon to view landmarks that would normally be covered
    • Isolation aperture drapes are large, clear plastic drapes with an adhesive backing surrounding the fenestration and are frequently used as drapes for hip pinning
    • The isolation drapes are used to drape a patient who has been positioned on a fracture table that maintains traction of the affected extremity
▶ Drape types
  » Each fenestrated drape has openings specific to the area to be exposed
    • Laparotomy or "lab sheet": abdomen
    • Pediatric or "pedi" sheet: pediatric abdomen
    • Transverse lap sheet: thorax and kidney

- Thyroid sheet: neck, especially the thyroid
- Extremity sheet: extremities
- Hip sheet: hip
- Perinea sheet: perineum
- Craniotomy sheet: cranium
  » Nonfenestrated sheets may be used to "square off" the surgical incision site, or to cover unaffected body parts that are not completely covered by the primary drape sheet
  » Nonfenestrated drapes are also custom designed to cover specific areas
  » Nonfenestrated split sheets are used to create an opening for a surgical site or to drape an extremity
  » Stockinettes are stretchable gauze tubes to cover extremities

STERILE PACKS

▶ Sterile packs are the first item opened for a surgical procedure and are placed onto the back table to serve as the initial sterile field
▶ Most basic sterile packs contain a Mayo stand cover, two gowns, a suture bag, four sticky paper drapes for square draping, and two paper towels for hand drying
  » General surgery: laparotomy pack; thyroidectomy pack
  » Gynecological surgery: vaginal hysterectomy pack; laparoscopy pack
  » Orthopedic surgery: arthroscopic pack; total hip pack
  » Genitourinary surgery: transurethral resection of the prostate (TURP) pack
  » Ear, nose, and throat surgery: ear pack
  » Neurosurgery: craniotomy pack
  » Cardiovascular surgery: coronary artery bypass grafting (CABG) pack
▶ Each specialized pack contains supplies and drapes that are specific to the specialty or the surgical procedure

SPONGES AND DRESSINGS

▶ Surgical sponges are used by the operative team to absorb blood and tissue fluids, for blunt dissection of tissues, and to protect important structures during the surgical procedure
▶ Surgical sponges are soft and lint free and contain a radiopaque strip so that they can be located by x-ray if left within a wound
▶ Laparotomy sponges (laps) are the largest and most absorbent of the surgical sponges and are available in several sizes, including small pediatric size (comes in packs of 5)
▶ Radiopaque four-by-fours (raytec sponges) are smaller and less absorbent than lap sponges. Used for procedures requiring smaller incisions. (Note: raytecs must never be used in open laparotomy cases unless they are put on the end of a sponge forceps.) (comes in packs of 10)
▶ Neurosurgical sponges are referred to as *patties* or cottonoids. Used to protect delicate neural tissue when suctioning and to assist with hemostasis during neurosurgical procedures (comes in packs of 10)
▶ Tonsil sponges are cotton-filled gauzes with a string attached, used during tonsillectomy to pack the bed after tonsil removal (comes in packs of 5)
▶ Kittner dissecting sponges are small rolls of cotton tape that are used to aid the surgeon in blunt dissection of tissues. Always loaded onto a clamp, such as a Rochester Pean (Kelly) for use (comes in a pack of 5). Note: They are also called "peanuts and dissectors."

Surgical Dressings

▶ A surgical dressing is applied to most wounds (traumatic or surgical) to serve the following functions:
  » Protect the wound from trauma
  » Protect the wound from microbial contamination
  » Absorb drainage and secretions
  » Support the incision
  » Provide pressure to reduce or eliminate dead space, reduce or prevent edema, assist in maintaining hemostasis, and prevent hematoma formation

» Maintain an environment that allows for preservation of new epithelial tissue and destruction of microbes

» Conceal the wound aesthetically

▶ In the OR, dressing application is considered the final step of the surgical procedure. Dressings must be applied using sterile technique. Dressing changes are also considered a sterile procedure

▶ Some dressing materials are referred to as sponges. Use caution not to confuse dressing sponges and surgical sponges (dressing sponges do not contain radiopaque markers)

▶ Dressing types determined by several factors

» Type, size, and location of wound

» Surgeon preference

» Age and size of the patient

» Underlying medical conditions (including known allergies)

» Condition of the surrounding skin

» Comfort of the patient

▶ Biologic dressings (biosynthetic skin substitutes)

» Used for temporary coverage of open wounds due to trauma, burns, or skin ulcers

• Integra

• Dermagraft

• Apligraf

▶ Skin graft: a graft that is surgically taken from a specific area of the patient's own body

» May come from another source such as from another person or may be obtained from a cadaver (homografts)

» Xenografts: heterografts involve tissue that is transplanted from one species to another (porcine, from pig)

▶ One-layer dressing

» Used to cover a small incision from which drainage is expected to be minimal

» Consists of transparent polyurethane film with an adhesive backing (Opsite, Bioclusive)

» Collodion: a type of liquid chemical dressing

» Dermabond: liquid skin adhesive applied by surgeons to close wounds

▶ Three-layer dressing

» Used to cover any size incision from which drainage (light, moderate, or heavy) is expected

» Inner (contact) layer: the wicking action of the contact layer allows passage of the drainage or secretions away from the healing wound into the intermediate absorbent layer

• Nonpermeable: mesh gauze

• Semipermeable: a hydrocolloid

• Permeable: non-adherent material (Telfa)

» Intermediate (absorbent) layer: placed over the contact layer to absorb any drainage or secretions (i.e., 4 × 4 gauze sponges)

» Outer (securing) layer: used to secure the contact and absorbent layers in position

• Tape: paper, silk, adhesive, cloth, foam

• Wrap: elastic bandage

• Stockinette: used prior to splint or cast application

• Tube gauze: used on a digit

• Montgomery straps: used in situations that may require frequent wound inspections or dressing changes

» Pressure dressing

• A type of three-layer dressing to which additional material is added to the intermediate layer or one that is tightly secured to cause compression of the surgical wound

• Immobilization of an area

• Support

• Absorption of excessive drainage

• Even pressure distribution

• Elimination of dead space

- Reduced edema
- Reduced hematoma formation
  » Bulky dressing
    - A type of three-layer dressing in which more material is added to the intermediate layer
    - Used to immobilize an area, provide additional support to the wound, and absorb excessive drainage
▶ Rigid dressings
  » Casts and splints are examples of rigid dressings applied following a closed traumatic injury or surgery to provide support and/or to prevent movement
    - Body jacket: extends from the axillae to the hips to immobilize the lower thoracic and lumbar vertebrae
    - Walking cast: cylindrical cast of the lower extremity that has a polyurethane sole or rubber heel added to allow for ambulation
    - Spica cast: secured to the torso to support the hip or shoulder in the desired position
    - Minerva jacket: extends from the head (incorporating the mandible while exposing the face) to the hips to immobilize the cervical and upper thoracic vertebrae
▶ Specialty dressings
  » Bolster dressing: sutured into position
  » Wet-to-dry dressing: gauze soaked in the liquid of surgeon's choice applied to wound and allowed to dry
  » Wet-to-wet dressing: wet dressing changed before it dries
  » Thyroid collar (Queen Anne's collar): circumferential neck wrap
  » Ostomy bag: applied over an intestinal stoma
  » Drain dressing: a Sof-Wick "y" shaped sponge to accommodate a wound that contains a drain
  » Tracheotomy dressing: dressing placed around a tracheotomy tube
  » Eye pad: oval-shaped gauze applied over the eyelid
  » Eye shield: rigid oval shield applied over the eye pad
  » Perineal (peri) pad: sanitary napkin
▶ Packing material
  » Used to assist with hemostasis, provide pressure, support a wound, and/or eliminate dead space
  » May be placed in the nose, rectum, vagina, or in an open wound

CATHETERS, TUBES, AND DRAINS
Catheters

▶ Used to remove fluid or other objects, such as thrombi and stones, from the body. They are also used to monitor body functions and for the instillation of fluids, including contrast media and medications
  » Urinary catheters: used to drain urine, but may have other applications as well
  » Robinson catheter: used to provide irrigation fluid within a duct or is threaded through the nasal cavity into the oral cavity and used to retract the uvula when a tonsillectomy is performed
  » Nonretaining catheters are temporarily inserted through the urethra into the bladder to obtain a urine specimen, decompress the bladder, or maneuver around an obstruction. They do not need a drainage bag attached
  » Foley catheters (indwelling urethral) used to measure urinary output over an extended period or provide bladder decompression. Uses a balloon to retain the catheter within the bladder
  » Suprapubic catheter: placed into the bladder through a surgical opening in the abdominal wall
  » Ureteral catheters: placed in the ureter(s) with the assistance of a cystoscope. Used to decompress the kidney, identify and protect the ureter(s) during pelvic procedures, and introduce contrast media during retrograde pyelography
▶ Intravascular catheters
  » Used to infuse fluids, obtain a diagnosis, monitor body functions, and remove thrombi

- » Venous access may be achieved peripherally, usually in the upper extremity, or centrally, for example, via the subclavian or jugular vein
- » Arterial catheters may be inserted temporarily to draw arterial blood for laboratory study or may be indwelling to provide information about the patient's physiological condition (i.e., arterial blood pressure)
- » A Fogarty is a balloon-tipped catheter: passed beyond an obstruction within the lumen of a vein, artery, or duct; balloon is inflated and the catheter is withdrawn along with the obstruction

Tubes

- ▶ Gastrointestinal tubes
  - » Used to aspirate air and fluids from the gastrointestinal tract
  - » May be passed through the nose or mouth into the stomach or intestine, through the rectum into the intestine, or may be inserted surgically (feeding tubes)
- ▶ Airway tubes
  - » Endotracheal (ET) tube: passed through the nose or mouth, between the vocal cords, and into the trachea of the unconscious patient
  - » Oral airway: inserted through the mouth to separate the jaws and depress the tongue
  - » Nasal airway: inserted through the nose to prevent obstruction of the airway due to relaxation of the soft palate (nasal "trumpet")
  - » Tracheotomy tube: placed directly into the trachea via an incision in the neck
- ▶ Chest tubes
  - » Inserted percutaneously through a "stab" wound to treat pneumothorax or following cardiothoracic surgical procedures to evacuate air and fluid from the pleural space

Drains

- ▶ Passive drains: allow a pathway for fluid or air to move from an area of high pressure to one of lower pressure
  - » Penrose drain: latex tubing that is placed partially within the wound, allowing fluid to move out of the wound into the dressing (capillary action)
  - » Cigarette drain: Penrose drain with gauze inside encourages fluid to move out of the wound into the dressing by wicking action
  - » T-tube: within the biliary system, it drains bile via gravity into a specialized collection unit called a bile bag
  - » Gastrostomy tube: inserted through the abdominal wall into the stomach; removes gastric contents or provides instillation of nourishment ("tube feeding")
  - » Cystostomy tube: inserted through the abdominal wall into the urinary bladder; removes urine
  - » Nephrostomy tube: inserted percutaneously into the kidney; removes urine
- ▶ Active drains: make use of negative pressure. Negative pressure is created by removing air from the collection device manually or mechanically
  - » Hemovac: typically used following orthopedic procedures when a moderate amount of drainage is expected
  - » Jackson-Pratt: used following abdominal procedures when a moderate amount of drainage is expected. Also used in neurosurgery and other general surgery procedures such as mammoplasty
  - » Stryker: used following orthopedic procedures; effective in reducing dead space due to the strength of the battery-operated evacuation pump

Chapter Review Questions

1. What kind of sterile surgical pack would be pulled for an orthopedic procedure?
   A. CABG pack
   B. Ear pack
   C. Laparotomy pack
   D. Arthroscopic pack

2. What kind of surgical sponges are referred to as *patties*?
   A. Lap sponges
   B. Cottonoids
   C. Raytec sponges
   D. Dressing sponges

3. Which one is *not* a function of the surgical dressing?
   A. Protect the wound from trauma
   B. Absorb drainage
   C. Remove air and fluids from the body
   D. Maintain an environment that allows for preservation of new epithelial tissue and destruction of microbes

4. What kind of dressing is used to cover a small incision from which drainage is expected to be minimal?
   A. One-layer dressing
   B. Three-layer dressing
   C. Bulky dressing
   D. Pressure dressing

5. What kind of catheter is used to measure urinary output over an extended period?
   A. Robinson red rubber catheter
   B. Coudé catheter
   C. Foley catheter
   D. Whistle catheter

6. What kind of airway tube is inserted through the nose to prevent obstruction of the airway due to relaxation of the soft palate?
   A. Endotracheal tube
   B. Nasal airway
   C. Tracheotomy tube
   D. Oral airway

7. A Penrose drain is considered
   A. A passive drain
   B. An active drain
   C. A Hemovac drain
   D. A Jackson-Pratt drain

8. How is a suprapubic catheter placed?
   A. In the ureter(s)
   B. Inserted temporarily to draw arterial blood for laboratory study
   C. Inserted into the lumen of a vein
   D. Into the bladder through a surgical opening in the abdominal wall

9. **What kind of dressing would you use for a thyroidectomy?**
    A. Ostomy bag
    B. Tracheotomy dressing
    C. Queen Anne's collar
    D. Bolster dressing

10. **What is another name for the Kittner sponges?**
    A. Peanut
    B. Dissector
    C. Sponge stick
    D. A and B

Answers

1. **D.** An Arthroscopic pack is pulled for an orthopedic procedure
2. **B.** The kind of surgical sponges that are referred to as "patties" are cottonoids
3. **C.** Protecting the wound from trauma; Absorb drainage; and maintaining an environment that allows for preservation of new epithelial tissue and destruction of microbes is all functions of a surgical dressing. Removing air and fluids from the body is NOT a function of surgical dressings.
4. **A.** The kind of dressing that is used to cover a small incision from which drainage is expected to be minimal is a One-layer dressing.
5. **C.** A Foley catheter is used to measure urinary output over an extended period.
6. **B.** A Nasal airway is a tube inserted through the nose to prevent obstruction of the airway due to relaxation of the soft palate.
7. **A.** A passive drain is a penrose drain.
8. **D.** A Suprapubic catheter is placed into the bladder through a surgical opening in the abdominal wall.
9. **C.** A Queen Anne's collar is used as a dressing for a Thyroidectomy.
10. **D.** A Peanut and a Dissector are other names for the Kittner sponges.

Reference

Association of Surgical Technologists. *Surgical Technology for the Surgical Technologist: A Positive Care Approach.* 4th ed. Boston: Delmar Cengage Learning.

11

Specialty Equipment

ENDOSCOPES

▶ Are used for diagnosis, biopsy, visualization, and/or repair of a structure within a body cavity or the interior of a hollow organ

▶ The endoscope is introduced either through a body opening, such as the urethra, or through a small skin incision

▶ Endoscopes can be attached to a camera that produces an image on a monitor for viewing by the surgical team

» Choledochoscopes: for exploration of the biliary system

» Mediastinoscopes: for visualization and biopsy of the structures of the mediastinum

» Ureteroscopes: for exploration of the ureters

» Angioscopes: for visualization of the heart and major vessels, or vascular endoscopes for the interior of smaller vessels

» Ventriculoscopes: for exploration of the brain's ventricular system

» Fetoscopes: for visualization of a fetus in utero

▶ Endoscopes can be used with electrosurgical devices for coagulation or tissue dissection

» Resectoscope uses a monopolar electric current to shave hypertrophied prostate tissue from within the proximal urethra, and instruments with monopolar cautery and bipolar electrosurgery active electrodes are commonly used during laparoscopy for tissue coagulation and dissection

POWERED INSTRUMENTS

▶ Instruments used in the OR that are powered by compressed air, nitrogen, electricity, or battery

» Drill holes into the skull and connect the holes to turn a bone flap for access to the brain

» Ream the central shaft of a long bone for rod placement

» Drill holes for screws to secure a plate on a fractured bone

» Saw the femoral or humeral head for joint replacement

» Saw through the sternum for access to the heart

» Reshape bone for plastic/reconstructive procedures

» Drive pins to reduce and stabilize fractured bone

» Cut skin, usually for skin grafting

» Sand the skin for dermabrasion

▶ Power saws have either a reciprocating (back and forth) or oscillating (side-to-side) action for cutting bone, and the blades for these power instruments are available in a variety of sizes and shapes

▶ Drills use a rapid rotary motion for carving bone with burs or drilling holes for wire, pins, or screws

▶ Reamers use a slower rotary motion for reaming the shaft of a long bone to insert a nail or rod
▶ Cranial perforators use a rotary motion to drill a hole in the cranium and are designed to stop before penetrating the brain
▶ Nitrogen for power instruments is supplied from a tank or is piped in from outside the surgery department
▶ Large power equipment is frequently powered by battery or nitrogen, whereas delicate bone work may require a faster air-powered instrument for greater precision and reduction of heat and vibration
▶ Many older dermatomes for skin grafts are electric powered, but the newer dermatomes and high-speed dermabraders are powered by compressed nitrogen

MICROSCOPES

▶ The compound operating microscope is a binocular apparatus that used bent light waves for variable magnification of tissues during microsurgery. It may be suspended from the ceiling or mounted on a mobile frame with locking casters
  » Magnification—the optical lens system provides the magnification and resolving power necessary to do the surgical work
  » Resolving power—refers to the ability of the optical system to filter out adjacent images and to clarify detail
  » Illumination—light waves for illumination of the operative field are provided by paraxial or coaxial illuminators
    • Paraxial illuminators contain tungsten or halogen bulbs and focusing lenses mounted to the body of the microscope and can be angled inward to illuminate the operative site
    • Coaxial illuminators use fiber optics to transmit light waves through the microscope's optical system. Light transmitted by this type of illuminator is cool to protect tissues from excessive heat

Video Monitors, Recorders, and Cameras

▶ Video cameras can be attached to microscopes or endoscopes so that the procedure can be viewed on a video monitor and recorded for documentation
▶ Video cameras should be sterilized according to the manufacturer's recommendations

Fiberoptic Headlamps and Light Sources

▶ Fiberoptic headlamps are worn by surgeons for additional lighting of the operative site
▶ Every specialty surgery makes use of the fiberoptic headlamp; it is most frequently worn by neurosurgeons, cardiovascular surgeons, and otorhinolaryngology surgeons
▶ To illuminate the interior of the body during endoscopic procedures, a fiberoptic light cord is connected to an electric light source at one end and to the endoscope at the other end

PULSE LAVAGE IRRIGATOR

▶ Powered by nitrogen, battery, or electricity and is used to thoroughly irrigate a traumatic, infected, or surgical wound
▶ It is often used during orthopedic procedures to irrigate contaminated fractures to clean out the debris and in total joint arthroplasties
▶ The surgical team must be protected from the splattered fluids, so a circular shield is often placed on the hand control

PHACOEMULSIFIER AND IRRIGATION/ASPIRATION UNITS

▶ Diseased eye lenses may be fragmented and removed with a phacoemulsifier, a machine that uses ultrasonic energy (cavitation) to fragment the lens, and an irrigator/aspirator (I/A) to remove the fragments
▶ The newer piezoelectric machine uses electric impulses to generate heat and is cooled by air or fluid that flows through the power cord

CRYOTHERAPY UNITS

▶ A cryotherapy unit uses liquid nitrogen, Freon, or carbon dioxide (CO_2) gas to deliver extreme cold through an insulated probe to diseased tissues, creating necrosis without damage to adjacent tissues
▶ Because cryotherapy preserves neighboring tissue and removes the diseased tissue without significant hemorrhage, it is useful for the removal of vascular tumors, brain tumors, and the prostate gland
▶ Cryotherapy is also used to repair retinal detachments and extract cataracts

INSUFFLATORS

▶ Laparoscopic procedures cannot be performed unless CO_2 gas is infused into the abdominal cavity through either a Veress insufflation needle or a Hasson blunt trocar
▶ Insufflator—machine that infuses CO_2 gas into the abdominal cavity
▶ Insufflation creates a space for viewing using an endoscope and for work within the cavity through cannulas inserted at strategic points through the abdominal wall
▶ The typical intraoperative pressure for laparoscopy is 12 to 15 mm Hg.

NERVE STIMULATORS

▶ Produce very small electric currents that, when applied to tissue, help to identify and preserve essential nerves for cranial, facial, neck, or hand reconstructive procedures
▶ The nerve stimulator is especially useful for identification of the seventh cranial (facial) nerve during acoustic neuroma removal and to identify the facial, acoustic, cochlear, and vestibular nerve branches during odontological procedures
▶ Anesthesia providers may use the nerve stimulator to access the actions of neuromuscular blockers administered during anesthesia

ACCESSORY EQUIPMENT

Suction Systems

▶ Suction apparatus uses a vacuum to remove fluids from the surgical site and patient's airway
▶ A minimum of two suction units is required in each operating room. One is for anesthesia, and the other is used within the surgical field
  » Vacuum source—may be portable or centralized
  » Vacuum source tubing—connects the vacuum source with the collection unit
  » Collection unit—may be reusable or contain a disposable liner
  » Tubing—connects the collection unit to the suction tip and is usually disposable
  » Suction tip—removes the fluid from the source

Lights

▶ White fluorescent overhead lights provide general illumination for the room
▶ Overhead operating lights are freely adjustable to any angle desired and provide an intense light appropriate for the size of the incision
▶ The light beam from the overhead OR light produces no shadows and minimal heat and is near the blue/white color of daylight

Pneumatic Tourniquets

▶ A tourniquet is used to restrict blood flow to the surgical site during some procedures
  » The amount of flood lost by the patient is minimized
  » Visualization of the surgical site for the sterile team members is improved
▶ Improper application of the tourniquet cuff may lead to blistering, bruising, pinching, or necrosis of the skin
▶ Cuff—consists of a rubber bladder contained within a fabric or plastic covering, similar to a blood pressure cuff (may be single or double chambers)
▶ Tubing—connects the cuff to the pressure source
▶ Pressure device—consists of an air compressor, pressure controls, pressure gauge, and timer

▶ Power source—the compressor is run by electricity, whether plugged into a wall or battery operated

▶ The surgeon is warned when the cuff has been inflated for 60 minutes and is then warned every 15 minutes after that time. The tourniquet is not allowed to be inflated for more than 90 minutes without being let down to allow tissues to be infused with blood supply

Sequential Compression Device (SCD)

▶ Consists of a compressor that is electrically operated, connecting tubing, and one or more sleeves that enclose that patient's limb(s)

▶ In the OR, SCDs are applied to the patient's legs to prevent venous stasis, thereby reducing the risk of development of deep vein thrombosis that can lead to pulmonary embolism

▶ SCDs are also used to treat edema and may be applied to the patient's upper extremity following an axillary lymph node dissection

Chapter Review Questions

1. What is used in surgery to restrict blood flow to the surgical site?
   A. Sequential compression devices
   B. Pneumatic tourniquets
   C. Insulators
   D. Suction

2. What is used for diagnosis, biopsy, visualization, and/or repair of a structure?
   A. Powered instruments
   B. Microscopes
   C. Endoscopes
   D. Phacoemulsifier

3. What kind of scope is used for exploration of the biliary system?
   A. Ventriculoscope
   B. Fetoscope
   C. Angioscope
   D. Choledochoscope

4. What action does a reciprocating saw have?
   A. Side-to-side
   B. Back-and-forth
   C. Rapid rotary motion
   D. Slow rotary motion

5. What is used in cranial, facial, neck, or hand reconstructive procedures to help identify and preserve essential nerves?
   A. Nerve stimulators
   B. Cryotherapy units
   C. Pulse lavage irrigator
   D. Pneumatic tourniquets

6. What is used in surgery to prevent deep vein thrombosis?
   A. Pneumatic tourniquets
   B. Endoscopes
   C. Cryotherapy units
   D. SCDs

7. What is a pulse lavage irrigator used for?
   A. To fragment and remove diseased eye lenses
   B. To help identify and preserve essential nerves
   C. To clean out traumatic or infected surgical wounds
   D. None of the above

8. Which one of the following is *not* accessory equipment?
   A. Suction
   B. Pneumatic tourniquet
   C. Sequential compression device
   D. Microscope

9. What is magnification?
   A. The ability of the optical system to filter out adjacent images and to clarify detail
   B. To view a surgical procedure on a video monitor and record for documentation
   C. Light waves for illumination of the operative field
   D. All of the selections are correct

10. **What scope is used to visualize a fetus in utero?**
    A. Choledochoscope
    B. Mediastinoscope
    C. Fetoscope
    D. Ureteroscope

Answers

1. **B.** Pneumatic tourniquets are used in surgery to restrict blood flow to the surgical site.
2. **C.** Endoscopes are used for diagnosis, biopsy, visualization, and/or repair of a structure.
3. **D.** The scope that is used for exploration of the biliary system is a Choledochoscope.
4. **B.** A reciprocating saw has a back-and-forth action.
5. **A.** A Nerve Stimulator is used in cranial, facial, neck, or hand reconstructive procedures to help identify and preserve essential nerves.
6. **D.** SCDs (sequential compression devices) are used in surgery to prevent deep vein thrombosis.
7. **C.** A pulse lavage irrigator is used to clean out traumatic or infected surgical wounds.
8. **D.** A Microscope is NOT an accessory equipment. A suction, pneumatic tourniquet and a sequential compression device are all considered to be an accessory equipment.
9. **A.** Magnification is the ability of the optical system to filter out adjacent images and to clarify details.
10. **C.** A Fetoscope is used to visualize a fetus in the uterus.

Reference

Association of Surgical Technologists. *Surgical Technology for the Surgical Technologist: A Positive Care Approach*. 4th ed. Boston, MA: Delmar Cengage Learning.

Intraoperative Procedures

12

Instrumentation

An understanding of design features can help in passing the right instrument at the right time, even if the surgeon does not specify the exact name of the instrument needed. The instrument is a tactile interface between the tissue and the surgeon's hands.

An instrument has several basic parts:

▶ Finger rings for precision
▶ Shank (long portion) of the instrument provide the tactile feedback needed for precision surgery
▶ Points or teeth—toothed or sharp-pointed instruments are used to grip fibrous tissue that would otherwise slip through the instrument's jaws. Forceps with smooth ridges along the tips, such as vascular forceps, are used to grasp more delicate tissue.

CLASSIFICATION/FUNCTION

▶ Clamping—any instrument that closes over tissue to hold or occlude it
  » *Example: hemostat*
▶ Thumb forceps—a nonlocking instrument used for grasping tissue and suture needles during suturing and for general tissue manipulation. They are also called "pickups"
  » *Example: Cushing forceps*
▶ Cutting instruments—Instruments used to cut or dissect various tissues
  » Scalpel blade—detachable from the knife handle. Used to make the incision
    • Blades are #10, #15, #11, #12, #15, #20, #23, Beaver blades
    • Knife handles (Figure 12.1):
      • #3 handle; #10, #15, #11, #12 blades
      • #7 and #9 handle: takes the same blades as the #3 handle
      • #4 handle: #20, #23 blades

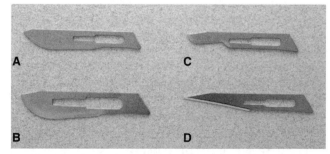

Figure 12.1 Surgical knife blades: **A.** #10 blade. **B.** #20 blade. **C.** #15 blade. **D.** #11 blade. (Reproduced with permission, from Hoffman B et al., eds. *Williams Gynecology*. 3rd ed. New York, NY: McGraw-Hill Education; 2016.)

» Scissors—used to dissect tissue
  • Small, sharp-tipped scissors, such as iris scissors, are used for extremely fine dissection in plastic surgery
  • Castroviejo scissors are commonly used in microsurgery
  • Round-tipped, light dissecting scissors, such as Metzenbaum scissors, are used extensively on delicate tissue in general surgery
  • Fibrous connective tissue requires heavier scissors, such as the curved Mayo scissors
  • Straight Mayo scissors are used for cutting suture and dressings
  • Wire-cutting scissors are used for stainless steel and other metal suture materials
» Rongeur—used to cut and extract tissue; distinguished by having a spring-loaded hinge
  • May have a single hinge (single-action rongeur) or two hinges (double-action rongeur)
» Shears—large cutting instruments used to sever bone tissue. Their most common use is during thoracic surgery when one or more ribs must be cut for access to the chest cavity
» Curette—a small cup with a sharpened, serrated, or smooth rim at the end of the handle
  • Very fine curettes are used in ear, paranasal, and spinal surgery
  • Larger, heavier curettes are used in orthopedic procedures
» Osteotome, chisel, and gouge
  • Chisel—an orthopedic cutting instrument that is used with a mallet (like chisels used in sculpting or carpentry)
  • Gouge—a V-shaped bone chisel
  • Osteotome—beveled on both sides. A large osteotome often is used to remove bone from the iliac crest for use as a graft elsewhere in the body
» Elevator—used to separate or "lift" tissue
  • Lambotte elevator slices tissue as it elevates
  • Key elevator has a sharp edge but is much more delicate
  • Penfield and Freer elevators are used in soft tissue surgery such as neural and vascular procedures
  • Joker has a short handle, and strong tip making it ideal for separating connective tissue layers without causing bleeding
» Rasp—used to remodel bone
» Saw—used in procedures that require bone cutting

RETRACTION INSTRUMENTS

Retraction instruments are used to hold back tissue layers.

▶ Handheld versus self-retaining
  » Handheld retractors range in size from the very fragile skin hook used in plastic surgery to the large, 4-inch (10-cm)-wide Deaver retractor used in abdominal procedures
  » Other common retractors are the Army-Navy retractor, vein retractor, Goelet retractor, and Richardson, ribbon, and Harrington ("sweetheart") retractors
  » The rake retractor generally is used only for connective tissue
  » Sharp rakes or hooks are designed to grasp the undersurface of superficial tissues
  » Small Senn retractor is used in plastic or superficial surgery
  » A commonly used instrument is the double-ended retractor
  » Self-retaining retractors hold tissue against the walls of the surgical wound by mechanical action. They can have many attachments suited to the needs of the surgery
    • The O'Sullivan-O'Connor, Bookwalter, and Balfour retractors are examples
    • Finochietto self-retaining retractor is used in cardiothoracic surgery
  » The smaller Gelpi and Weitlaner retractors are used for superficial incisions
  » McPherson self-retaining lid speculum is used to retract the eyelids

DILATORS AND PROBING INSTRUMENTS

▶ Dilator—a cylindrical instrument used to increase the inside diameter of a tubular structure

▶ Delicate dilators are used in tear duct surgery, whereas the larger cervical dilators are used to dilate the cervix so that instruments can be passed into the uterus

▶ Urethral dilators are used to open a stricture of the urethra

MEASURING INSTRUMENTS

▶ A uterine sound is inserted into the cervix to measure the depth of the uterus from the cervix to the fundus

▶ Orthopedic calipers are used to prepare the bone for a joint implant. A depth gauge is used in orthopedic surgery to determine the length of screws to be implanted into bone

▶ A sizer is a trial, reusable replica of an implantable prosthesis. A sizer allows the surgeon to test a replica first

  » *Example: before a cardiac valve is inserted, a sizer is used to determine the correct size*

SUTURING INSTRUMENTS

▶ A needle holder is used to grasp a curved needle during suturing. The length, weight, and type of tip must be matched to the suture and tissue

  » Heaney or May-Hagar needle holder is considered a heavy needle holder
    • Usually these needle holders will hold an SH needle and bigger

  » Sharp-tipped needle holder, such as the Sarot needle holder, is used for fine sutures (i.e., 4-0 and smaller)

  » Lightweight or fine-tipped needle holder (e.g., the Webster needle holder) does not have enough surface area at the tip to grasp a heavy needle

SURGICAL STAPLING AND LIGATING DEVICES

▶ Are used to perform multiple suture and resection maneuvers. Staplers are available as single-use medical devices or as stainless steel instruments

▶ Several manufacturers make surgical stapling instruments

  » Skin stapler—places a single line of staples across the incision border and is used for closing a skin incision

  » Gastrointestinal anastomosis (GIA)—places a double row containing two staples in each row and severs the tissue between rows when fired

  » Ligating-dividing stapler (LDS)—places a double row containing two staples in each row and severs the tissue between rows when fired

  » Circular or end-to-end anastomosis (EEA) stapler—used for end-to-end intestinal resection (cutting and rejoining). It joins two arms of intestine with a double row of staples

  » Thoracoabdominal (TA) stapler—has a right-angled firing section that fits around deep structures for resection and anastomosis. It is commonly used in lung or abdominal surgery

  » Purse-string stapler—performs the same function as a purse-string suture and places circumferential nylon sutures and staples

▶ Hemostatic clips

  » V-shaped staples that close down and occlude a vessel or duct

  » Small, medium, and large clips are available in cartridges that are color-coded by size

  » Pass the clip applier with the tip down, taking care not to squeeze the handles, which would release the clip prematurely

SUCTION INSTRUMENTS

▶ Suction (aspiration) is needed during a surgical procedure to clear blood, fluids, and small bits of tissue debris from the surgical site and provide an unobstructed view of the anatomy

▶ Poole suction—the tip is designed for abdominal surgery and has a removable perforated guard that protects bowel and intestinal organs from injury by spreading the suction pressure over many small holes in the guard

▶ The Yankauer or tonsil suction tip is designed to suction in the chest cavity and throat

▶ Frazier tip is designed to suction in superficial areas in the face, neck, and ear and in neurological and some peripheral vascular procedures (many Frazier tips will come with an obturator to clear out the lumen of the suction tip)

APPLICATION: USE OF INSTRUMENTS BY TISSUE TYPE

▶ Skin is incised rather than cut with scissors. This is because the elastic quality of skin makes it difficult to cut an exact straight line with scissors

▶ Visceral serosa, or organs of the body, are covered by a fine membrane called the serosa. This membrane is easily punctured, and the underlying tissue layers can bleed profusely. Therefore, atraumatic instruments are needed when handling this tissue

▶ Lung, spleen, liver, thyroid—these highly vascular tissues are very delicate, bleed profusely, tear easily, and have little or no elasticity. Only partially occluding clamps ad smooth tissue forceps are used on the tissues

  » When the spleen, liver, and intestines are retracted, the retractor blade must be sufficiently wide to distribute the pressure. A wide Deaver, Richardson, or Harrington retractor is often used for liver and spleen

  » Lung tissue is held with broad-tipped, partially occluding clamps such as the Duval lung clamp

▶ Peritoneum—the lining of the body cavities is smooth, elastic, and strong. Normal peritoneal tissue is dissected with Metzenbaum scissors (the most commonly used scissors in general surgery) and may be grasped with toothed forceps or Allis clamps

▶ Adipose tissue—loose connective tissue, such as the subcutaneous tissue of the abdomen, has a high fat content. Adipose tissue has few blood vessels compared with other types of tissue. This allows the use of penetrating retractors, such as a sharp rake or Weitlaner (self-retaining). The Allis clamp, which has a T tip with fine serrations at the tip, often is used to clamp or grasp adipose tissue. Toothed forceps are used for suturing adipose tissue

▶ Muscle—striated muscle tissue is moved aside or the muscle bundles are manually separated rather than cut whenever possible during surgery. Large muscles are elastic and fibrous, allowing for the use of toothed forceps and clamps

▶ Bone—bone tissue is resilient and somewhat springy

  » Large bones are manipulated using traction or leverage rather than direct pulling

  » Bone retractors, such as the Bennett and Scoville retractors, have a toothed tip or a reverse curve that can be inserted under another bone for leverage. The Lewin clamp wraps around bone for manual traction

▶ Cartilage, tendon, and fascia—these are extremely strong and resilient. These tissues can be quite slippery, requiring toothed clamps or those with ridges to maintain the hold

  » Tendons are covered by a sheath that is strong and smooth. Kocher clamps can handle this tissue. Martin clamps have double rows of heavy teeth and are frequently used in knee surgery for grasping the medial and lateral tendons

  » Fascia is grasped with Kocher clamps. Strong dissecting scissors such as curved Mayo scissors are used on fascia and large tendons

Chapter Review Questions

1. Which clamp would be used for a thyroidectomy?
   A. Kocher
   B. Babcock
   C. Lahey
   D. Heaney

2. Which retractor would most likely be used for gynecologic surgery?
   A. Finochietto
   B. Bookwalter
   C. Balfour
   D. O'Connor-O'Sullivan

3. A non-crushing clamp used to grasp the mesoappendix is a/an
   A. hemostat.
   B. Babcock.
   C. Kelly.
   D. Allis.

4. What scissors are used on vascular procedures on vessels?
   A. Metzenbaum
   B. Jacobson
   C. Potts-Smith
   D. Stevens

5. All of the following are handheld retractors except
   A. Army-Navy.
   B. Deaver.
   C. Heiss.
   D. Harrington.

6. What is a gouge?
   A. A V-shaped bone chisel
   B. A hinged instrument with sharp, cup-shaped tips that is used to extract pieces of bone or other connective tissue
   C. An orthopedic instrument used to slice bone; one side is straight and the other is beveled
   D. A straight instrument with curved sharp or dull tip used to separate tissue layers such as periosteum from bone

7. What kind of blade can be placed on a #4 knife handle?
   A. #10
   B. #11
   C. #20
   D. #15

8. Which one is considered a cutting instrument?
   A. Curette
   B. Balfour
   C. Osteotome
   D. A and C

9. **What is used to remodel bone?**
    A. Elevator
    B. Dilator
    C. GIA stapler
    D. Rasp

10. **What type of instrument is used on the visceral serosa?**
    A. Toothed, hooked, or serrated instruments
    B. Atraumatic instruments
    C. Sharp rakes and Allis clamps
    D. Toothed forceps

Answers

1. **C.** A Lahey clamp is used to grasp the thyroid
2. **D.** O'Connor-O'Sullivan retractor is used in gynecologic surgery
3. **B.** Babcock
4. **C.** Potts-Smith scissors
5. **C.** A Heiss retractor is a self retaining retractor
6. **A.** A V-shaped bone chisel
7. **C.** #20
8. **D.** A and C
9. **D.** Rasp
10. **B.** Atraumatic instruments

Reference

Fuller J. *Surgical Technology: Principles and Practice*. 6th ed. Philadelphia, PA: Saunders.

13

Surgical Procedures

SURGICAL INCISIONS

Provide access to the operative site, allow maximum exposure, and ease of extension, while keeping wound closure and cosmesis in mind (Figure 13.1).

▶ Midline
  » Vertical midline—preferred for most abdominal surgeries
  » Easily extended superiorly and inferiorly
  » Provides maximum exposure and allows rapid access
  » Can be used for almost every region of the abdominal cavity and retroperitoneum
  » Upper midline—"above the midline"—used for esophageal hiatus, stomach, spleen and pancreatic surgery
▶ Paramedian—vertical incisions placed either to the left or right of the midline on the abdominal wall
▶ Subcostal (Kocher)
  » Right—for exposure of the gallbladder and biliary tree
  » Left—for splenectomy
▶ McBurney—obliquely placed, muscle-splitting right iliac fossa incision used for appendectomy
▶ Rockey-Davis—similar to McBurney incision, oriented transversely, allows for better cosmesis
▶ Inguinal—lower oblique
▶ Pfannenstiel—for access to the retropubic space. The incision is placed in the interspinous crease above the symphysis pubis. Most commonly used for gynecologic procedures.
▶ Midabdominal Transverse—Horizontal Flank
▶ Thoracoabdominal—for access to upper abdominal organs
  » Left—for access to the left hemidiaphragm, gastroesophageal junction, distal pancreas and left kidney
  » Right—access to the right hemidiaphragm, esophagus, liver, inferior vena cava and right kidney.
▶ Transverse

GENERAL SURGERY

Laparoscopic Surgery—General Considerations

Many procedure are performed laparoscopically. The goal of laparoscopic surgery is to perform the procedure in the same manner while optimizing the outcome for the patient. Benefits to the patient may include:

▶ Decreased pain from smaller incisions
▶ Decreased hospital and recovery time
▶ Quicker return to activities of daily living and work

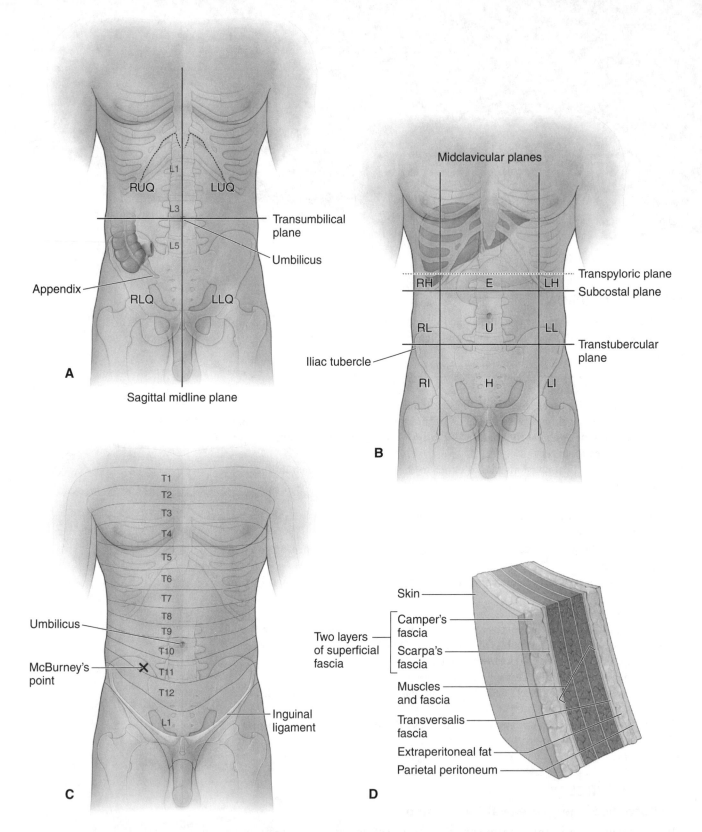

Figure 13.1 Abdominal cavity layers. **A.** Quadrant partitioning: right upper quadrant (RUQ); left upper quadrant (LUQ); right lower quadrant (RLQ); and left lower quadrant (LLQ). **B.** Regional partitioning: right hypochondriac (RH); right lumbar (RL); right iliac (RI); epigastrium (E); umbilical (U); hypogastrium (H); left hypochondriac (LH); left lumbar (LL); and left iliac (LI). **C.** Surface anatomy and dermatome levels. **D.** Fascial layers of the anterior abdominal wall. (Reproduced, with permission, from Morton DA, Foreman KB, Albertine KH. *Gross Anatomy: The Big Picture.* New York, NY: McGraw-Hill Education; 2011.)

Laparoscopic or minimal invasive (MIS) surgery is performed using minimal access with the creation of a pneumoperitoneum. The following steps can be applied to the beginning of basic laparoscopic general, gynecologic, and urologic surgery procedures.

▶ Pneumoperitoneum is created with carbon dioxide gas, either with an open technique or by closed needle technique.
▶ A small incision is made in the upper edge of the umbilicus.
  » The closed technique consist of a special hollow insufflation needle (Veress needle) that is spring-loaded with a retractable cutting outer sheath. It is inserted into the peritoneal cavity and used for insufflation of the carbon dioxide gas.
  » Open technique consists of a supraumbilical incision through the fascia and into the peritoneal cavity. A blunt cannula (Hasson cannula) is inserted into the peritoneal cavity and anchored to the fascia with 2-0 Polyglactin 910 suture.
▶ Once an adequate pneumoperitoneum is established (intra-abdominal pressure 12–15 mm Hg), a 10-mm trocar is inserted through the supraumbilical incision. The laparoscope with the attached video camera is passed through the umbilical port and the abdomen inspected.

Appendectomy

▶ Right lower quadrant incision made at McBurney's point
▶ After entry into the abdominal cavity slight Trendelenburg position can be used with a tilt to patient's left
▶ The cecum is used to assist in location of appendix
▶ Mesentery of appendix is divided to allow exposure of the base of appendix
▶ The stump is ligated and mucosa is obliterated with the cautery

Laparoscopic Appendectomy

▶ Visualization similar to open appendectomy with the use of three ports/trocars
▶ Base of appendix is stapled along with the mesentery, or clipped or cauterized
▶ The appendix is removed via a retrieval bag

Bariatric Surgery

▶ Produce weight loss through restriction of intake and malabsorption of ingested food
▶ Roux-en-Y gastric bypass is the most common procedure performed
  » A separate small gastric pouch is created from the proximal stomach and connected to a segment of proximal jejunum
▶ The gastric sleeve-narrows the stomach by anastomotic stapling

Breast Surgery

▶ Diagnostic features to accompany breast surgery
  » Needle localization
  » Fine needle aspiration
  » Sentinel lymph node biopsy or dissection
    • Used to assess the regional lymph nodes for axillary lymph-node metastases
    • Gamma probe is used with the injection of isosulfan blue or methylene blue for visualization
▶ Excisional biopsy—removal of breast lesion with margin of normal-appearing breast tissue
▶ Breast-conserving procedures for carcinoma involve resection of the breast cancer with a margin of normal-appearing breast tissue. Additional therapy may be required. No axillary lymph node dissection is performed.
  » Segmental mastectomy
  » Lumpectomy
  » Partial mastectomy
  » Wide local excision
▶ Mastectomy with axillary dissection
  » Skin-sparing mastectomy that removes all breast tissue, the nipple-areola complex
▶ Total (simple) mastectomy—removes all breast tissue, the nipple-areola complex and skin

The intra-abdominal pressure must not exceed 15 mm Hg. Increased pressure may cause risk of pulmonary embolism.

▶ Extended simple mastectomy—removes all breast tissue, the nipple-areola complex, skin and level I axillary lymph nodes

▶ Modified radical mastectomy—removes all breast tissue, the nipple-areola complex, skin and level I, II, and III axillary lymph nodes

Cholecystectomy

Laparoscopic Cholecystectomy

▶ Performed the same way as an open procedure

▶ Following placement of trocars and camera:
  » The fundus of the gallbladder is grasped and retracted cephalad
  » An additional grasper is used to expose the triangle of Calot.
  » Cystic duct is dissected free and clipped at the cystic duct–gallbladder junction
  » For a cholangiogram—a small opening is made in the cystic duct to allow cholangiogram catheter insertion
  » The cystic duct is divided, then the cystic artery clipped and divided, allowing for removal of the gallbladder via trocar

Open Cholecystectomy

▶ Performed infrequently. May be done as a conversion to open procedure or if deemed necessary during a laparotomy (exploratory procedure)

Colon Resections

Performed for neoplasms, inflammatory bowel disease, obstruction, and perforation.

For most colon and bowel resections patient will be in the supine position. Noted exceptions are the low anterior resection and sigmoid resection where access to the anus and rectum is needed. These patients will be positioned in lithotomy position.

Instrumentation for colon and small bowel resection include:

▶ Major abdominal sets with long instrumentation
  » Kelly clamps
  » Mixter
  » Babcock
▶ Handheld retractors
  » Richardson
  » Deaver
  » Harrington
▶ Self-retaining retractor Bookwalter or Balfour

Types of Colon Resection (Figure 13.2)

▶ Right colectomy—for lesions or disease of the right colon

▶ Transverse colectomy—for lesions in the mid and distal transverse colon

▶ Left colectomy—for lesions of the distal transverse colon, splenic flexure, or descending colon

▶ Sigmoid colectomy—for lesions of the sigmoid colon, entire mobilization of the splenic flexure if required for anastomosis

▶ Total and subtotal—for colitis

▶ Low anterior resection—for lesions of the upper and mid rectum (circular stapling device is used for anastomosis)

▶ Colostomy—surgical creation of an opening in the colon which is then brought to the an opening in the skin (stoma) (Figure 13.3)
  » Preoperative marking of the stoma is ideal for patient quality-of-life issues
  » Should be located within the rectus muscle, away from bony prominences, abdominal creases, and previous scars

Small Bowel Resection

▶ Performed for small bowel obstructions
  » Adhesions
  » Tumors
  » Hernia

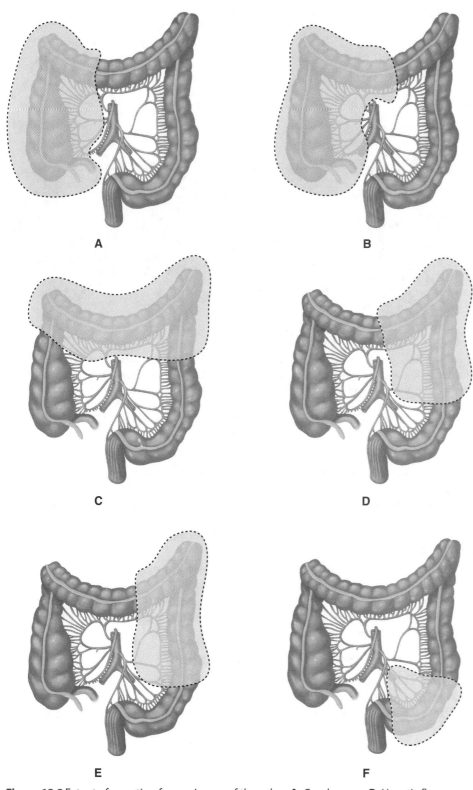

Figure 13.2 Extent of resection for carcinoma of the colon. **A.** Cecal cancer. **B.** Hepatic flexure cancer. **C.** Transverse colon cancer. **D.** Splenic flexure cancer. **E.** Descending colon cancer. **F.** Sigmoid colon cancer. (Reproduced, with permission, from Brunicardi FC et al, eds. *Schwartz's Principles of Surgery*. 10th ed. New York, NY: McGraw-Hill Education; 2014.)

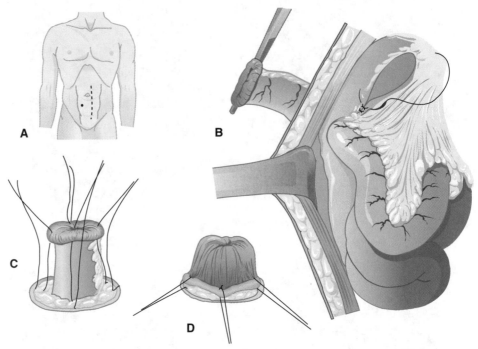

Figure 13.3 Ileostomy after colectomy. **A.** A midline incision for colectomy is indicated by the dotted line and the site of the ileostomy by the black dot. **B.** The ileum has been brought through the abdominal wall. **C, D.** The ileostomy stoma has been everted and its margins sutured to the edges of the wound. (Reproduced, with permission, from Doherty GM, ed. *CURRENT Diagnosis & Treatment Surgery*. 14th ed. New York, NY: McGraw-Hill Education; 2015.)

► Affected intestine is examined for viability, color, peristalsis, and marginal arterial pulsations
► Nonviable bowel is resected and an end-to-end anastomosis is performed on viable portion

Meckel's Diverticulum

► Usually found in the ileum within 100 cm of the ileocecal valve
► Failure or incomplete vitelline duct obliteration
► Segmental resection of ileum that includes the diverticulum is performed
► Ileostomy—surgical creation of an opening in the ilium that is then brought to the an opening in the skin (stoma)

Esophagectomy and Partial Esophageal Resection

► Performed for cancer, stricture, or dysplastic mucosal changes
► Thoracic approach is probable depending on site
► Removal of diseased portion of esophagus and portion of stomach depending on site of tumor
► Reconstruction and end-to-end anastomosis probable with stomach, jejunum, or colon

Gastrectomy

Perform for carcinoma.

► Procedures
  » Gastric bypass
  » Partial gastrectomy
  » Gastroduodenostomy
  » Billroth I—distal gastrectomy (at the antrum of the stomach) with reconstruction to connect the gastric remnant to the duodenum via anastomosis
  » Gastrojejunostomy-permanent communication between the proximal jejunum and the stomach

» Billroth II—distal gastrectomy along with reconstruction to connect the gastric remnant to the jejunum via anastomosis

Gastrostomy

▶ Creation of an opening into the stomach through the skin for relief of blockage or for nutritional purposes.

Hemorrhoidectomy

▶ Removal of hemorrhoids—submucosal tissue of the anal canal that contains venules, arterioles and smooth muscle fibers
▶ Treated by rubber band ligation or submucosal resection
  » Submucosal resection includes:
    • The patient in jackknife position
    • Fansler anoscope for exposure and addition rectal retractors
    • Minor instrument set
    • Packing

Hernia

▶ An area of weakness or complete disruption of the fibromuscular tissues for the body wall.
▶ Structures arising from the cavity contained by the body wall can pass through, or herniated, through such a defect
▶ Refers to the actual anatomic weakness or defect, and hernia contents describe those structures that pass through the defect.
▶ Surgical repair of the inguinal hernia is the most common general surgery procedure performed today.
▶ More common in males than females
▶ Congenital, abdominal wall hernias include
  » Umbilical
  » Epigastric
  » Inguinal
  » Femoral
  » Spigelian
  » Obturator
  » Sciatic
  » Lumbar
  » Perineal
▶ Congenital internal hernias or postoperative hernias include
  » Incisional
  » Ostomy-related
  » Mesenteric defects
▶ Direct—located within Hesselbach's triangle
  » Are acquired
  » Thought to develop from an acquired weakness in the fibromuscular structures of the inguinal floor
▶ Femoral—located caudal or inferior to the inguinal ligament in a medial position
▶ Indirect—lateral to the inferior epigastric vessels
▶ Inguinal hernia:
  » Indirect: hernias that develop lateral to the inferior epigastric vessels.
  » Develops at the site of the internal ring, or the spermatic cord in men.
  » In women, develop where the round ligament enters the abdomen.
  » Indirect inguinal hernias are thought to be congenital in etiology.
▶ Operative Techniques:
  » Shouldice technique: commonly used for open repair of inguinal hernias and is the most popular pure tissue hernia repair
  » Cooper ligament repair: the only technique that definitively repairs both the inguinal and femoral hernia defects in the groin

» Polypropylene mesh is the most common prosthetic used today in mesh repairs of the inguinal hernia. The two most common prosthetic repairs are the Lichtenstein and the "plug and patch" repair.
  • Lichtenstein technique: the first pure prosthetic, tension-free repair to achieve consistently low recurrence rates in long-term outcomes analysis
» Preperitoneal approach (done laparoscopically)—this approach is more effective than the traditional anterior herniorrhaphy because a repair in the preperitoneal

Hepatic Resection

▶ Usually performed for hepatic cysts, benign liver lesions, malignant liver tumors
▶ Right subcostal incision with possible partial or complete left subcostal extension across the midline
▶ Instruments include:
  » Fixed table retractor (e.g., Thompson or Bookwalter)
  » Abdominal instrument sets with long instruments
▶ Additional supplies include intraoperative ultrasound
▶ A cholecystectomy may be performed

Liver Transplant

▶ Removal of a diseased organ, surgically replacing it with a donor organ
▶ Disease process can be from chronic liver disease or cirrhosis

Radiofrequency Ablation

▶ For treatment of liver tumors
▶ Radiofrequency (RF) waves deliver an alternating electric current that pass through living tissue without causing pain or neuromuscular excitation
▶ The resistance of the tissue to the rapidly alternating current produced heat
▶ Can be performed in a minimally invasive approach or via laparotomy

Nissen Fundoplication

▶ Primary antireflux repair
▶ Usually performed laparoscopically
▶ The distal esophagus is mobilized, the crura is closed, and the posterior aspect of the gastric fundus is wrapped around the esophagus and secured with 2-0 nonabsorbable sutures

Pilonidal Cystectomy

▶ Pilonidal disease consists of a cyst/infection of a hair-containing sinus or abscess occurring in the intergluteal cleft
▶ Acute abscess requires incision and drainage
▶ Patient is in the prone position
▶ Procedures involve unroofing the sinus tract, curetting the case, and marsupializing the wound
▶ Z-plasty, advancement flap, or rotational flap may be required with extensive resections

Pyloromyotomy

▶ An incision made through the pyloric muscle to release a stricture or stenosis

Splenectomy

▶ Surgical removal of the spleen
▶ Patient positioned in the supine position
▶ Left subcostal incision used for elective procedure
▶ Midline incision optimal for exposure in ruptured spleen or enlarged spleen procedures
▶ Laparoscopic approach may be used in elective procedures

Vagotomy

▶ A resection of a portion of the vagus nerve
▶ Performed to tread peptic ulcer disease

Whipple Procedure—Pancreaticoduodenectomy

▶ Performed for pancreatic carcinoma
▶ Removal of the head of the pancreas, duodenum, portion of the jejunum, the distal third of the stomach, and lower half of the common bile duct including removal of gallbladder
▶ Uses a midline incision from xiphoid to umbilicus or bilateral subcostal incisions

GENITOURINARY SURGERY

Adrenalectomy

▶ Removal of the adrenal gland(s)
▶ Performed for adenomas
▶ Laparoscopic adrenalectomy is preferred. Laparotomy is performed for large tumors
▶ Bilateral adrenalectomy is performed for patients with adrenal hyperplasia
▶ Confirm the position with the surgeon as the approach may be anterior, lateral, or posterior via retroperitoneum

Circumcision

▶ Surgical removal of the prepuce of the penis
▶ Performed for religious and cultural reasons (often performed on infants)
▶ Also performed on with infection, phimosis, or paraphimosis

Hypospadias Repair

▶ Performed to correct the urethral meatus opening on the ventral side of the penis proximal to the tip of the glans penis

Kidney Transplant

▶ May be from a cadaver or living donor
▶ Living donor nephrectomy is preformed laparoscopically
▶ Performed due to renal disease such as end-stage renal disease
▶ Are usually placed in the iliac fossa because of the proximity to the recipient's bladder and iliac vessels

Nephrectomy

▶ Removal of a kidney
▶ Performed for carcinoma, chronic infections, nonfunctioning kidneys, and symptomatic polycystic kidney disease
▶ Laparoscopic or open approach can be used
▶ The specimen can be retrieved via a specimen bag and laparoscopic port made larger to allow removal
▶ The Hand Assisted Laparoscopy technique (HAL) may also be used
▶ Patients are positioned in a lateral kidney position (Figure 13.4)

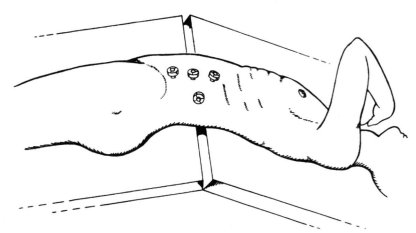

Figure 13.4 One of the possible port configurations for left retroperitoneal laparoscopic nephrectomy. (Reproduced, with permission, from McAninch JW, Lue TF. *Smith and Tanagho's General Urology.* 18th ed. New York, NY: McGraw-Hill Education; 2012.)

Orchiectomy

▶ Removal of one or both testes due to carcinoma
  » Simple orchiectomy removes the testicle and epididymis
  » Radical orchiectomy removes the hemiscrotum, tunica vaginalis, and spermatic cord

Orchiopexy

▶ A fixation of the testis in the scrotal sac.
▶ Procedure performed for torsion of the testicle or spermatic cord, undescended testis

Prostatectomy

▶ Performed for prostate carcinoma
▶ Radical prostatectomy
  » Seminal vesicles, prostate, and ampullae of the vas deferens are removed
  » Can be performed open retropubic, transperineal, or laparoscopic; with or without robotic assistance

Vasectomy

▶ Excision of a section of the vas deferens for the purpose of permanent sterilization

Cystectomy

Removal of bladder or portion of bladder (depending of type and site of cancer)

▶ Radical cystectomy
  » In men—removal of the bladder, prostate, and seminal vesicles
  » In women—removal of the bladder, cervix, uterus, anterior vaginal vault, urethra and ovaries

ENDOSCOPIC UROLOGIC PROCEDURES

Cystoscopy

▶ Endoscopic inspection of the lower urinary tract
▶ Patient is placed in the lithotomy position in stirrups
▶ Equipment required:
  » Sterile irrigation
  » Fiberoptic light cord
  » Rigid cystoscope and flexible cystoscopes
  » Working port
  » Video cameras are attached to the optical eyepiece of the cystoscope

Transurethral Resection of the Prostrate

▶ Removal of prostate tissue through endoscopic means using a resectoscope designed to excise, fulgurate, or vaporize tissue
▶ Performed for benign prostatic hypertrophy (BPH)
▶ Endo resection loops are used to remove the prostate tissue

Ureteroscopy

▶ Performed to visualize the ureters
▶ Used for management of ureteral occlusion, treatment of ureteral calculi, and placement of ureteral stents

OBSTETRIC AND GYNECOLOGIC SURGERY

For the following procedures:

▶ The patient may be in supine (laparotomy) or lithotomy position (laparoscopic)
▶ An abdominal prep with vaginal prep may be used. The frog-leg position is used to perform the prep and insert a Foley catheter when the procedure will be in supine position

Diagnostic Laparoscopy

▶ A minimally invasive option for evaluation of the pelvic and abdominal organs
▶ Commonly performed to evaluate pelvic pain, causes of infertility, endometriosis, adhesions, and pelvic masses

Dilatation and Curettage (D & C or D & E)

The patient is positioned in lithotomy position using stirrups

▶ A rigid cannula attached to an electric-powered vacuum empties the uterus
▶ May be accompanied by sharp curettage
▶ The cervix is first dilated
▶ The pregnancy or retained product of conception are evacuated by suction—suction curettage—or by mechanically scraping out the contents—sharp curettage, or both.

Ovarian Cystectomy

▶ Ovarian cyst excision. Removal of cyst alone or with reconstruction of ovary to limit postoperative adhesions
▶ Minimal invasive approach (laparoscopic) versus laparotomy depending on reconstruction
▶ Incisional choice is Pfannenstiel incision

Salpingo-oophorectomy

▶ Removal of the ovary and fallopian tube
▶ Laparoscopic approach performed unless malignancy is suspected
▶ Laterality needs to be determined

Oophorectomy

▶ Surgical removal of ovary

Tubal Sterilization

▶ Tubal ligation
  » Midtubal segment of fallopian tube is excised
  » Done when laparoscopy is not an option for the patient
  » Parkland and Pomeroy techniques are used
▶ Laparoscopic tubal sterilization methods
  » Filshie clip—applied via metal applicator that houses the clip; the clip locks around the tube
  » Bipolar electrosurgical coagulation—current is applied to the tubes until completely desiccated in a section
  » Silastic band—applied with aid of a custom metal applicator that draws the tube up and allows the band be pushed down onto the tube
  » Hulka clip—a spring loaded clip that is loaded into a metal applicator and held in the unlocked position until placed around the tube and locked into place
▶ Salpingectomy
  » A midtubal segment of fallopian tube is cauterized or removed
  » Often performed laparoscopically
▶ Salpingostomy
  » A lengthwise linear incision of the fallopian tube

Abdominal Myomectomy

▶ Surgical removal of leiomyomas from surrounding myometrium
▶ Performed to preserve the uterus and for those of childbearing age
▶ Indications include abnormal uterine bleeding, pelvic pain, and infertility
▶ Often performed via laparotomy, although can be performed laparoscopically
▶ Uterine tourniquet is applied to occlude both the uterine and ovarian vessels
▶ Serosal Pitressin injection is used to limit uterine blood loss
▶ Sharp and blunt dissection of the surrounding the leiomyoma is used to free the tumor from the adjacent myometrium

Abdominal Hysterectomy

▶ One of the most common gynecologic procedures preformed
▶ Performed for symptomatic leiomyomas, pelvic organ prolapse, adenomyosis, endometriosis, chronic pain, premalignant or cervical disease
▶ Performed through an abdominal transverse or vertical incision
▶ May be performed laparoscopically and robotically
  » Total hysterectomy includes the removal of uterus and cervix. Bilateral salpingo-oophorectomy (BSO) may be included
  » Supracervical hysterectomy includes the removal of uterus above the cervix
▶ The patient is positioned in supine position
▶ Transverse or vertical incision is used

Vaginal Hysterectomy

▶ Performed for uterine prolapse, benign disease, relatively small uterus, and when adhesions are not anticipated
▶ Patients usually have decreased pain and hospital stay
▶ Patient is positioned in lithotomy position
▶ A Foley catheter is inserted during the vaginal prep
▶ The surgeon requires a draped instrument tray and additional drape for the lap while seated for procedure
▶ Vasopressin solution or 0.5% lidocaine with epinephrine solution may injected at the incision
▶ Instruments include Auvard weighted vaginal speculum, right-angle retractor, and vaginal hysterectomy tray
▶ Specialty items include vaginal packing and cream with a perineal pad for dressing

Laparoscopic Assisted Vaginal Hysterectomy (LAVH)

▶ The ureters are identified
▶ Proximal round ligament is grasped and divided along with the broad ligament
▶ Vesicouterine fold is elevated away from the underlying bladder and incised
▶ Uterine arteries are coagulated and transected from a vaginal approach
▶ The uterus is delivered vaginally
▶ Vaginal vault is closed
▶ The pelvis is re-insufflated and examined via the laparoscope

Trachelectomy

▶ Removal of the cervix
▶ For women who have had a supracervical hysterectomy and present with vault prolapse, persistent cyclic bleeding, or preinvasive cervical lesions
▶ Similar to a vaginal hysterectomy, although entry into the peritoneal cavity is not necessary since the cervical cuff lies outside the cavity
▶ Patient is positioned in the lithotomy position and a Foley is inserted

Hysteroscopy

▶ Allows endoscopic view of the endometrial cavity and tubal ostia
▶ Performed for abnormal uterine bleeding, infertility, or identified uterine cavity mass
▶ Contraindications include pregnancy and current reproductive tract infection
▶ A single-toothed tenaculum is placed on the anterior cervical lip
▶ Distention medium flow begins and the hysteroscope is introduced into the endocervical canal
▶ Resection is performed
▶ Care must be taken to monitor the input and output of all fluid

Bartholin Gland Duct Cyst

▶ Cyst or abscess resulting from ductal opening obstruction followed by accumulation of mucus or pus with the gland duct
▶ Marsupialization or I & D is performed
▶ Cultures can be taken of any fluid

Cesarean Delivery (C-Section)

▶ Indications for a cesarean delivery include fetal distress, breech or other malpresentation, triplet and higher order gestations, cephalopelvic disproportion, failure to progress, placenta previa, or active genital herpes
▶ Abdominal access is usually gained through a Pfannenstiel incision
▶ Uterine incision may be vertical or transverse
▶ The baby is delivered with speed, the umbilical cord is clamped and cut and baby is handed off the sterile field to the gowned neonatologist or pediatrician, the placenta is delivered
▶ Bleeding is controlled and closure begins immediately

Cervical Conization

▶ Removes ectocervical lesions and a portion of the endocervical canal by means of a conical tissue biopsy
▶ An effective means of treating carcinoma in situ and adenocarcinoma in situ
▶ Procedures include
  » Cold knife conization
  » LEEP (loop endocervical electrocautery procedure)
  » Laser

Cervical Cerclage

▶ Shirodkar procedure
  » For an incompetent cervical os
  » Placement of a heavy surgical suture tape around the cervix to prevent spontaneous abortion

Retropubic Urethropexy

  » Burch and Marshall-Marchetti-Krantz colposuspension procedures
  » Suspend and anchor the pubocervical fascia to the musculoskeletal framework of the pelvis
  » For treatment of stress urinary incontinence (SUI)

OTORHINOLARYNGOLOGIC SURGERY

Myringotomy

▶ Tympanostomy tubes are placed to aerate the middle ear space and prevent accumulation of middle ear inflammation and effusion

Tonsillectomy and Adenoidectomy

▶ Most common operations performed on children
▶ Performed for recurrent streptococcal tonsillitis and airway obstruction
▶ Often performed in combination
▶ Tonsillectomy—procedure involves an incision of the mucosa adjacent to the tonsil along with anterior pillar, identification of the tonsillar capsule, and subcapsular dissection of the tonsil free from the underlying muscle bed
▶ Adenoidectomy—removal of the adenoid tissue

Uvulopalatopharyngoplasty (UPPP)

▶ Treatment for sleep apnea
▶ Conservative excision of the inferior margin of the soft palate, uvula, excision of redundant mucosa with suture fixation of the pharynx and palate
▶ Tonsillectomy is also performed

Laser-Assisted Uvuloplasty (LAUP)

▶ Treatment of sleep apnea
▶ Inferior margin of the soft palate and uvula are excised using laser (CO_2)

Glossectomy

▶ Resection of the tongue
▶ Procedure performed for carcinoma

Obstetrics Terms

Lightening—the settling of the fetal head into the brim of the pelvis

Gravida—the total number of pregnancies that a women has had, regardless of outcome

Parity—the number of births

Quickening—maternal perception of movement

APGAR scores—reflect the cardio-respiratory and neurologic status at 1 and 5 minutes of life

Hemiglossectomy

▶ Partial resection of the tongue
▶ Performed for carcinoma
▶ Tongue reduction for sleep apnea

Thyroidectomy

▶ Removal of the thyroid gland, total or partial (right or left lobe)
▶ Performed for malignant tumors, cysts larger than 4 cm
▶ Total thyroidectomy is usually recommended
▶ Partial thyroidectomy or lobectomy may be performed
▶ A completion thyroidectomy is performed if a diagnosis of malignancy is made

Parathyroidectomy

▶ Removal of the parathyroid glands
▶ Performed for primary hyperparathyroidism

Tracheotomy

▶ An incision into the trachea

Tracheostomy

▶ An incision into the trachea in which a tube can be placed for the patient to breathe
▶ For prolonged intubation and airway management

Radical Neck Dissection

▶ An en bloc removal of all nodal groups between the mandible and the clavicle for carcinoma including:
  » Sternocleidomastoid muscle
  » Internal jugular vein
  » The spinal accessory nerve
▶ Supplies include:
  » Nerve stimulator
  » Vessel loops
  » Small vascular clamps and instruments available
  » "Peanut" dissectors

Parotidectomy

▶ Removal of the parotid gland
▶ Removed with a radical neck dissection
▶ Nerve stimulator for facial nerve identification used

Scalene Node Biopsy

▶ For diagnosis of intrathoracic neoplasms
▶ Inferior deep cervical nodes that lie in the supraclavicular fossa behind the sternocleidomastoid muscle, easily biopsied

Septoplasty

▶ To correct cartilaginous or bony abnormalities of the septum such as septal deviation

Turbinectomy

▶ Resection of the nasal turbinates, may be done in conjunction with other procedures

Functional Endoscopic Surgery (FESS)

▶ Uses fiberoptic and small endoscopes to visualize the paranasal sinuses
▶ Preserves sinonasal mucosa
▶ Mucosal polyps can be debrided carefully
▶ Enlarges the natural ostia
▶ Ethmoid sinuses are unroofed

Endoscopic Procedures
▶ Bronchoscopy—rigid, for removal of foreign body or tracheal dilatation or biopsy
▶ Esophagoscopy—rigid, performed to rule out esophageal perforation
▶ Laryngoscopy—direct visualization of the larynx
▶ Microlaryngoscopy for examination of the vocal cords and treatment of nodules

PLASTIC SURGERY

Rhytidectomy
▶ "Facelift"—the procedure performed for the aging face
▶ Characteristics of the aging face may include:
  » Brow ptosis
  » Deepening of nasolabial fold
  » Decent of the mid-face

Minifacelift
▶ "Minilift" is the procedure performed on those with limited skin laxity
▶ Advantages include less risk to the facial nerve and shorter recovery time
▶ Disadvantages include limited access to the facial nerve and difficulty visualizing for hemostasis
▶ Types of minifacelifts include
  » Short scar lift
  » Minimal access cranial suspension lift

> Knowledge of the anatomy of the facial nerve is essential to avoiding nerve injury. The frontal and marginal branches are the most commonly injured branches in facelift.

Browlift
▶ May be done in conjunction with a blepharoplasty and rhytidectomy or as separate procedure
▶ Two most common browlifts performed
  » Coronal—open with incision hidden above the hairline
    • Involves making a large incision approximately 4–6 cm posterior to the hairline and elevating subgaleally down to the brow. Once all the tissues are released, the brow is then suspended in a more superior direction.
  » Endoscopic—4 to 5 small incisions hidden above the hairline
    • The brow is released widely and the periosteum and galea are secured to the skull using a variety of drill-assisted securing techniques and devices. As compared to the coronal browlift, the endoscopic approach does not require excision of hair-bearing skin while still allowing the surgeon to widely release the tissues necessary to achieve long-term brow elevation.

Midface Lift
▶ Intended to resuspend the cheek prominence and decrease the depth of the nasolabial crease

Blepharoplasty (Eye Lift)
Upper Blepharoplasty
▶ Skin excision follows the natural lid crease
▶ 8–12 mm above the ciliary margin along the upper edge of the tarsal plate
▶ The incision extends medially to an area above the level of the medial canthus
▶ Superior incision is determined by the amount of skin to be incised
▶ Hemostasis is achieved using bipolar cautery

Lower Blepharoplasty
▶ Can be approached using several techniques
  » Skin flap—addresses fat and skin
  » Skin-muscle flap—addresses fat, muscle, and skin
  » Transconjunctival—addresses the orbital fat
▶ Conjunctiva is anesthetized with topical tetracaine. Direct injection of local anesthetic is used for surrounding tissue. Protection of the globe is vital with the use of a shield

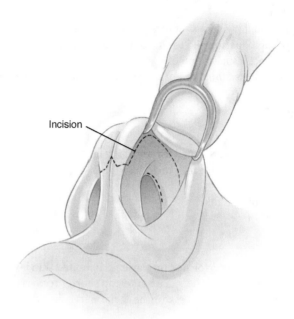

Incision

Figure 13.5 Incisions used for rhinoplasty—transcolumellar, marginal, and intercartilaginous. (Reproduced, with permission, from Lalwani AK, ed. *CURRENT Diagnosis & Treatment in Otolaryngology—Head & Neck Surgery.* 3rd ed. New York, NY: McGraw-Hill Education; 2011.)

Rhinoplasty

▶ Rhinoplasty surgery addresses the bony and cartilaginous dorsum, nasal valves, tip, and nasal base (Figure 13.5)
▶ Incisions used include:
  » Intercartilaginous
  » Marginal
  » Transcolumellar
▶ May be performed under sedation or general anesthesia
▶ Approaches include:
  » Open/external
  » Closed
  » Endonasal
▶ Cocaine pledgets are placed intranasal against the septum after induction of anesthesia
▶ 1% Lidocaine with Epinephrine 1:100,000 in injected regionally
▶ Septum is usually the first choice for graft-ear cartilage is often the second choice if the septum is not adequate

Skin Grafts

Detaches epidermis and varying amounts of dermis from its blood supply in the donor area; graft is placed in a new area known as the recipient area

▶ Split-thickness grafts
  » Are thin, usually the epidermis and possibly a slight bit of the dermis
  » Donor sites heal rapidly
  » Can be meshed to expand (Dermatome and Mesher)
▶ Full thickness
  » Include the epidermis and all of the dermis
  » Most aesthetically desirable of free grafts, least contracture
  » Donor sites include postauricular, supraclavicular, antecubical, inguinal, and genital area
▶ Biological skin substitutes
  » Sources vary (porcine, human)
    • Bovine collagen used to mimic human dermal layer of skin
    • Chemically prepared cadaver skin

Cartilage graft may be taken from the septum, ear, or rib. An alternate site may be needed to be prepped and draped out for this graft site.

Breast Reconstruction

▶ The implantation of a prosthesis or autologous tissue
▶ Some autologous tissue flaps include
  » TRAM—transverse rectus abdominis myocutaneous—supplied by the deep superior and inferior epigastric vessels
  » Latissimus dorsi—supplied by the thoracodorsal vessels
  » DIEP flap—deep inferior epigastric perforator flap—unlike the TRAM, this flap spares the muscle

Breast Augmentation

▶ To increase the size of the breast
▶ May be accompanied by mastopexy (lifting of the breast) correction of asymmetry
▶ Silicone bag is filled with sterile saline solution or silicone and placed beneath the breast tissue either in the submammary or subpectoral plane
▶ Subareolar, inframammary fold, or axillary incisions may be used

Reduction Mammoplasty

▶ Decrease the size of the breast due to mammary hyperplasia
  » Patients experience back and shoulder pain
▶ Breast tissue is removed and breast are reconstructed
▶ Breast tissue is sent to the laboratory for examination
▶ Suction-assisted lipectomy (SAL) may be used during the procedure
▶ Additional supplies include:
  » Scale to weigh breast tissue
  » SAL catheters, tubing and machine
  » Tumescent solution, pump tubing

SAL Suction-Assisted Lipectomy/Liposuction

▶ Tissue is infiltrated with tumescent solution
  » 1 mg of epinephrine (1:1000) and 250 mg of lidocaine (1%) per 1000 mL of Ringer's lactate solution
▶ A small cannula is introduced through a small incision and suction is applied with a suction machine
▶ The fat layer enlarged by the tumescent solution dislodges and is able to be suctioned, eliminating abnormal bulges or localized fat

Gynecomastia

▶ Male breast excess
▶ Removal includes liposuction and subcutaneous mastectomy

Otoplasty

▶ Procedure to correct prominauris (prominent ears)

Mentoplasty

▶ Chin augmentation
▶ Can be implanted via external or intraoral route

Cleft Lip Repair

▶ Repair of the cleft that may involve the floor of the nostril and lip on one or both sides and may extend through the alveolus
▶ May be in combination with a cleft palate

Cleft Palate

▶ Repair of the hard and soft palate
▶ Goals:
  » To repair both the nasal and oral mucosa
  » To repair the levator muscle in the soft palate

DENTAL PROCEDURES

With all dental procedures, especially fractures, airway precautions are a priority.

Le Fort I Fractures (Figure 13.6)

▶ Fractures that separate the palate from the midface, result in a mobile palate but a stable upper midface
▶ Procedure involves reducing the facture by aligning the dentition into as normal a configuration as possible

Le Fort II Fractures (Figure 13.6)

▶ Fractures involve the frontonasal maxillary buttress, and often the skull base via the ethmoid bone
▶ This fracture has a pyramidal appearance and results in palatal and upper-midface mobility
▶ Nasotracheal intubation should be avoided
  » Procedure involves alignment of dentition using arch bars and wires or screws to reduce the fracture (intermaxillary fixation).

Le Fort III Fractures (Figure 13.6)

▶ Involves the same structures as Le Fort II fractures, but fractures have occurred with greater degree of force
▶ This fracture also includes the frontozygomatic buttress, resulting in complete craniofacial dislocations
▶ Associated neurological injuries are often seen in these patients
▶ Intermaxillary fixation is performed, along with repair of frontozygomatic buttress and zygomatic arch and plating of the lower maxilla

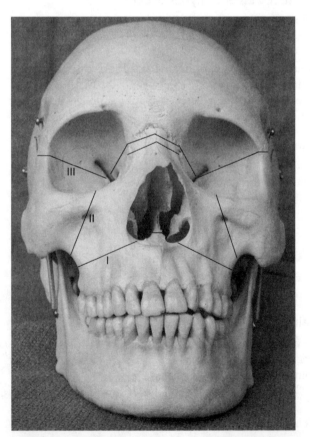

Figure 13.6 Anterior view of Le Fort midface fractures. (Reproduced, with permission, from Lalwani AK, ed. *CURRENT Diagnosis & Treatment in Otolaryngology—Head & Neck Surgery*. 3rd ed. New York, NY: McGraw-Hill Education; 2011.)

Mandible Fractures

▶ May occur as a result of sports activities, falls, motor vehicle accidents, or interpersonal trauma
▶ Open rigid fixation techniques utilize titanium plates and screws and allow primary bone healing due to compression of the bone fracture segments
▶ Airway precautions are a priority with these patients

OPHTHALMOLOGIC SURGERY

Case Planning

▶ Psychological considerations: Although many patients look forward to correcting medical problems to improve or restore their eyesight, they often have unspoken fears that a poor outcome will result in blindness
▶ Verification of the operative site: The team must be especially vigilant during the Time Out of this surgery
▶ Positioning: This surgery is performed with the patient in the supine position with the head stabilized on a circular headrest (sometimes called a doughnut)
▶ Prepping and draping: The standard approved eye prep antisepsis is dilute povidone-iodine (5% or as directed by the surgeon). A number of techniques are used to drape the eye, but it is important to isolate the hairline and nonoperative side of the face
▶ Anesthesia: Most ophthalmic surgery is performed using a regional anesthetic with monitored sedation. A topical anesthetic, local infiltration, peribulbar nerve block, or a combination of these is most often used
▶ Ophthalmic drugs: Ophthalmic surgery requires the use of many types of drugs that are administered preoperatively, during surgery, and in the postoperative period. Many of these drugs have potent effects, and a medication error could irreparably damage the eye
  » Drugs that dilate the pupil (mydriatics)
  » Drugs that paralyze accommodation and inhibit focusing (cycloplegics)
  » Miotics
  » Topical anesthetics
  » Injectable anesthetics
  » Additives to local anesthetics
  » Viscoelastics
  » Viscoadherents
  » Irrigants
  » Hyperosmotic agents
  » Anti-inflammatory agents
  » Anti-infective drugs
  » Other drugs: cocaine, mitomycin, dextrose, etc.
▶ Instruments: Ophthalmic instruments are delicate and expensive. The most important thing about these instruments is keeping the tips very clean
  » Sharp items must be smooth, and scissor blades must align properly
  » Needle holders are particularly susceptible to injury; the scrub should make sure that catches an spring mechanisms are working properly
  » Suction tips must be checked for patency

Surgical Procedures

▶ Excision of a chalazion: nodal tissue arising from a sebaceous gland is excised from the tarsal plate
▶ Repair of an entropion: an abnormal inversion of the lower eyelid
▶ Repair of an ectropion: drooping of the lower eyelid
▶ Excision of a pterygium: the pterygium membrane is surgically removed to prevent loss of vision. It is a patch of degenerative elastic tissue that proliferates from the conjunctiva in response to chronic irritation
▶ Dacryocystorhinostomy: the creation of a permanent opening in the tear duct for the drainage of tears
▶ Lacrimal duct probing: the lacrimal duct is opened and an obstruction is removed

▶ Muscle resection and recession: performed to correct deviation of the eye caused by strabismus (a condition in which the eyes are unable to focus on point because the muscles lack coordination)

▶ Penetrating keratoplasty (corneal transplantation): a full-thickness transplantation of a donor cornea to restore vison

▶ Lasik (laser-assisted in situ keratomileusis): performed to shape the curvature of the cornea and correct a refractive problem

▶ Extracapsular cataract extraction (phacoemulsification): the fragmentation of tissue by ultrasonic vibration

▶ Anterior vitrectomy: performed to remove the vitreous from the anterior chamber

▶ Scleral buckling procedure for detached retina: performed when the sensory layer of the retina becomes separated from the pigment epithelial layer

▶ Trabeculectomy: performed to create a channel from which the aqueous humor may drain from the anterior chamber. This procedure is performed for the treatment of glaucoma

▶ Argon laser trabeculoplasty: the argon laser is used to shrink collagen and stretch the canal of Schlemm, thereby expanding the canal, increasing drainage, and reducing IOP (intraocular pressure)

▶ Orbital decompression: one or more bony sections of the orbital cavity are removed to reduce pressure on the optic nerve. This is often performed to treat hyperthyroidism (Graves disease)

▶ Enucleation: a complete removal of the eyeball (globe). Evisceration is a similar procedure in which the contents of the eye are removed, but the outer shell of the sclera and the muscle attachments are left intact

▶ Orbital exenteration: the removal of the entire eye and orbital contents including the eyelids, ocular muscles, and orbital fat. This procedure is performed for the treatment of cancer

ORTHOPEDIC SURGERY

Positioning

Patients are positioned for orthopedic surgery on the standard operating table or on a specialty table. The modern orthopedic table also called the *fracture table* is used mainly for surgery of the femur and lower leg.

Classification of Fractures

▶ Name of the bone and location: name of bone and location
▶ Pattern of the fracture: pattern of break
  » Transverse: the fracture line is perpendicular to the long axis of the bone
  » Oblique: a type of transverse fracture that occurs at an angle
  » Spiral: a fracture of the long bone that occurs in a spiral pattern as the result of twisting or torsion on the bone
  » Impacted: a fracture in which bone fragments are driven into each other or into another bone
  » Comminuted: a fracture with two or more pieces
  » Open: a fracture in which the fractured end penetrates the skin
  » Greenstick: a fracture of immature bone that is soft and less brittle than mature bone (common in pediatric patients)
  » Depressed: refers to cranial fracture in which the fragments are displaced
  » Level of comminution: extent of fracture
  » Displacement: describes whether the bone fragments are in anatomical alignment
  » Pathologic origin: a pathologic fracture occurring with normal load
▶ Internal fixation: requires surgery to insert or implant a device that holds the bone fragments in place (metal plates, rods, pins and screws)
▶ External fixation: a means of stabilizing bone fragments in anatomical position from outside the body

Arthroscopic Surgery

A minimally invasive surgery (MIS) of the joints. This technique is used mainly for diagnostic procedures and for repair and reconstruction of soft tissue

▶ Bankart procedure

▶ Open rotator cuff repair
▶ Elbow arthroplasty
▶ Carpal tunnel release

Surgical Approaches to the Hip and Pelvis

▶ Intramedullary femoral nailing: a femoral nail is a rigid rod that is seated in the medullary canal and held in position with locking screws placed at a 90-degree angle to the nail
▶ Hip arthroplasty: performed to replace diseased components of the hip joint, including the acetabulum, trochanter, and ball of the femur, with one or more artificial implants
▶ Surgical fixation of the pelvis: performed to reduce and stabilize and fractured pelvis

Surgical Approaches to the Knee and Lower Leg

▶ Knee arthroscopy: a common technique for assessing and correcting problems arising from injury and disease
  » Arthroscopic meniscectomy: a tear in the meniscus is the most common knee injury. Complete meniscectomy leaves the medial rim of the structure to share load bearing and stabilize the knee
  » Arthroscopic anterior cruciate ligament (ACL) repair: repair of the ACL routinely is performed arthroscopically. A graft is taken from the central portion of the patellar tendon to replace the torn ACL
▶ Knee arthroplasty: performed to relieve pain and allow the patient to resume activity. This procedure can be arthroscopically or open. It can also be a total knee replacement or a partial knee replacement
▶ Intramedullary nailing (tibia): an intramedullary rod (nail) is inserted into the tibia for fixation and stabilization of a fracture

Surgical Approaches to the Foot

▶ Repair of the Achilles tendon: performed to return strength and flexibility to the foot after a traumatic injury. A posterolateral approach is used and the incision is made parallel to the tendon on the lateral or median ide with a #15 knife blade
▶ Triple arthrodesis: fusion of the talocalcaneal, talonavicular, and calcaneocuboid joints. Performed by removing the cartilage from each joint and allowing them to heal in approximation. The surgical goal is to prevent movement of these joints and thereby prevent pain and joint instability
▶ Fracture of the ankle: Open reduction and internal fixation of the foot is performed to stabilize fractures of the distal tibia, fibula, talus, and calcaneus. Performed using cannulated screws, pins, wires, and plates
▶ Bunionectomy: performed to alleviate pain and increase patient mobility. In a bunionectomy, an enlarged metatarsal head (hallux valgus) is reduced or removed
▶ Hammertoe correction: this is a condition in which a toe has contracted at the proximal interphalangeal joint, the middle joint in the toe. Contracture of the ligaments and tendons causes the toes to curl downward. Hammertoe may occur in any toe except the big toe.

VASCULAR SURGERY

Techniques

▶ Endarterectomy: the removal of atherosclerotic plaque from the inside of the artery
▶ Vessel anastomosis: longitudinal or circumferential incisions in the blood vessel are closed with a double-arm suture. Traction sutures may be placed at one or both ends of the incision
▶ Graft tunneling: vascular grafts often must be tunneled through subcutaneous tissue or other layers to connect one vessel to another. The surgeon may use the fingers to separate the tissue digitally, or a graft tunneler can be used

Surgical Procedures

▶ Intraoperative angiography: the injection of contrast medium into a selected artery and its branches to determine the exact location of strictures, occlusion, or malformations. During surgery, intraoperative angiography is use in conjunction with angioplasty to allow the surgeon to see the position of the stricture and to place the catheter in the correct location

▶ Transluminal angioplasty: the insertion of an arterial catheter or stent into an artery to establish patency and normal blood flow

▶ Insertion of a vena cava filter: a vena cava filter is a metal, umbrella-shaped filter inserted into the inferior vena cava to prevent emboli from entering the pulmonary system. The filter can be temporary or permanent

▶ Vascular access for renal hemodialysis: An anastomosis between the arterial and venous systems is created surgically to produce access, on a long-term basis, to the vascular system. This is for patients with severe or end-stage renal disease

▶ Thrombectomy (open procedure): to remove a stationary clot in a blood vessel. Commonly performed with an embolectomy catheter

▶ Carotid endarterectomy: the surgical removal of atherosclerotic plaque from the carotid artery

▶ Abdominal aortic aneurysm (AAA): a condition in which a section of the abdominal aorta becomes thin and bulges because of atherosclerotic plaque and progressive weakening of the aortic wall. The repair of an abdominal aortic aneurysm can be performed via an open abdominal or endovascular approach

▶ Aortofemoral bypass: performed to treat aortoiliac occlusive disease

▶ Axillofemoral bypass: creates circulation between the femoral arteries and the axillary artery. This restores circulation to the lower extremity or, in an emergency procedure, bypasses an infected aortic graft or aneurysm

▶ Femorofemoral bypass: involves implantation of a prosthetic graft that connects the femoral artery on the affected side to the opposite femoral artery. This is done to bypass unilateral atherosclerotic disease in the iliac artery

▶ In situ saphenous femoropopliteal bypass: a surgical alternative to the use of a synthetic graft to bypass a diseased femoral artery. The saphenous vein is not removed but is left in anatomical position. This is usually done when the bypass has to go past the knee joint.

▶ Femoropopliteal bypass: a synthetic graft or autograft is implanted between the femoral and popliteal arteries

▶ Saphenous vein graft: the greater saphenous vein is removed to provide an autograft for peripheral or coronary artery bypass

▶ Management of varicose veins: involves the removal of dilated and tortuous (varicose) veins and their tributaries to prevent symptoms and to improve cosmetic appearance

▶ Above-the-knee-amputation: surgical removal of the leg. Performed when vascular insufficiency caused by arteriosclerotic or thrombotic disease results in necrosis of the lower limb

CARDIOTHORACIC SURGERY

Thoracic Surgery

The most difficult part of any Cardiothoracic surgery will be in learning the set up. Everything else is handled in phases.

▶ Thoracoscopic lung biopsy: Endoscopic removal of lung tissue for pathologic assessment

▶ Lung volume reduction: portions of the lung severely affected by chronic pulmonary emphysema are removed to improve pulmonary function

▶ Scalene node biopsy: performed on patients with palpable nodes in the area of the scalene fat pads. Biopsy is performed to establish cancer staging or to confirm a diagnosis

▶ Thoracotomy: the general term for open surgery of the thoracic cavity

▶ Lobectomy: a lobe of the lung is removed to prevent the spread of cancer or to treat a benign tumor. Lobectomy may be performed as a VATS procedure or as an open procedure

▶ Pneumonectomy: the removal of the entire lung. (No chest tube is required in this procedure.)

▶ Rib resection for thoracic outlet syndrome (TOS), a rare condition in which the subclavian vessels and the brachial plexus are compressed at the apex of the thorax

▶ Decortication of the lung: the surgical removal of a portion of the parietal pleura. Chronic inflammation infection (empyema or tuberculosis) or a lung tumor causes the formation of exudates in the pleural space

▶ Lung transplantation: transplantation of one or both lungs is performed to remove a diseased lung and replace it with a donor lung

Cardiac Surgery

▶ Positioning: Procedures of the heart and associated structures are performed with the patient in the supine or lateral position with the affected side up.
▶ Incisions:
  » Median sternotomy (supine): a partial or full midline incision is made through the sternum
  » Paramedian (supine) incision is made to the right or left of sternum
  » Anterolateral, posterolateral: this is modification of the lateral position
  » Mini-thoracotomy (supine): the 2-inch (5-cm) right or left mini-thoracotomy is made between the ribs for access during minimally invasive and robotic procedures
▶ Surgical procedures:
  » Median sternotomy: a midline incision used for surgical procedures of the heart and great vessels in the thoracic cavity
  » Cardiopulmonary bypass: this mechanical bypass diverts blood away from the heart and lungs so that surgery can be performed
  » Sump catheterization: A sump catheter is inserted into the left ventricle soon after cardiopulmonary bypass has been established to suction blood and air and maintain cardiac decompression. By venting air, a sump catheter reduces the risk of air embolism in the systemic circulation
  » Infusion of a cardioplegic solution: this solution is used to stop the heart; this reduces the energy required by the cardiac muscle by elimination the energy requirements of contraction
  » Coronary artery bypass grafting (CABG) of a narrow segment of one or more coronary arteries is performed to improve circulation to the heart muscles
  » Transmyocardial revascularization (TMR): a series of small-bore transmural channels that are created with the carbon dioxide or holmium-yttrium-aluminum-garnet (holmium:YAG) laser to perfuse the myocardium
  » Resection of a left ventricular aneurysm: reduces the risk of rupture and embolism. Aneurysm is often caused by a reduced blood supply from an infracted coronary artery
  » Aortic valve replacement: replacement of a diseased valve. Common causes of valve insufficiency are endocarditis, congenital anomalies, and calcification
  » Mitral valve repair and replacement: a diseased mitral valve is replaced to open a constricted valve (stenosis) or to prevent blood from regurgitating into the left atrium. The valve is repaired with an annuloplasty; if the valve is severely damaged, it is replaced
  » Resection of an aneurysm of the ascending aorta: such an aneurysm can rupture or prevent the aortic valve leaflets from closing properly. The goal of resection of an aneurysm of the ascending aorta is to repair the aneurysm and restore function to the valve
  » Resection of an aneurysm of the aortic arch: such an aneurysm can impair blood flow to the brain and the upper body because of the frequent involvement of the aortic branches (i.e., the brachiocephalic artery, the left carotid artery, and the left subclavian artery, aka "great vessels")
  » Resection of an aneurysm of the descending thoracic aorta: performed to prevent rupture and life-threatening hemorrhage
  » Endovascular repair of a thoracic aneurysm: now frequently used for the treatment of descending thoracic aortic aneurysm (DTAA)
  » Insertion of an artificial cardiac pacemaker: implanted in the body to correct cardiac arrhythmia caused by a disease of the conduction system. A pulse generator provides electrical impulses through the device's cardiac leads, which are implanted in the conductive tissue of the heart
  » Replacement of a pacemaker battery: a malfunctioning pacemaker generator is replaced to produce continuous pacing
  » Implantable cardioverter-defibrillator (ICD): defibrillating and monitoring device used in patients susceptible to ventricular tachycardia or ventricular fibrillation
  » Surgery for atrial fibrillation (cardiac ablation): selective destruction of diseased conductive tissue to correct atrial fibrillation

» Pericardial window: accumulated blood or fluid in the pericardium can compress the heart and impede filling of the ventricles. This reduces the amount of blood ejected into the systemic circulation. Removal of the fluid, through the creation of a pericardial window, improves cardiac function
» Pericardiectomy: chronic inflammation of the pericardium can produce a fibrotic (and often calcified) coating over the heart that constricts the ventricles. Removal of the adherent scar tissue improves cardiac function.

▶ Heart failure techniques:
» Insertion and removal of an intra-aortic balloon catheter (IAB): reduces the workload of the heart after myocardial infarction or in patients who cannot be taken off bypass
» Ventricular assist device (VAD): used to wean patients from cardiopulmonary bypass when other means are ineffective. Patients awaiting heart transplantation also may be candidates for a VAD, which consist of a polyurethane blood sac, flexible diaphragm, and pump assembly
» Heart transplantation: may be performed in suitable patients with end-stage cardiac disease

Video-Assisted Thoracic Surgery (VATS)

Minimally invasive surgery of the thoracic cavity.

▶ Case planning:
» Patient preparation: the patient is placed in the lateral position with the operative side up and a general anesthetic is administered through a double-lumen endotracheal tube
» Trocar and cannulas: endoscopic ports are placed according to the procedure. Three or four ports usually are required
» Instruments: thoracoscopy in an adult requires 10-mm lenses, 0 and 30 degrees. The scope, camera, and light source are managed as for all minimally invasive endoscopic procedures. The thoracoscopy instruments are the same as regular instruments, but they are put on long handles and can fit in a port (trocar/sheath)

NEUROLOGIC SURGERY

Positioning

▶ For cranial procedures, the surgeon and assistant stand at the patient's head and the scrub stands to the surgeon's right or at the overhead table
▶ During spinal procedures, a right-handed surgeon usually stands at the patient's left side and the assistant stands on the patient's right side. The scrub should stand to the patient's left unless otherwise directed
▶ Peripheral nerve procedures on a patient's upper extremities may be performed with the surgical team seated around a hand table
▶ Team positioning during procedures with the patient in the high Fowler position may need to be altered to accommodate standing platforms for scrubbed personnel to ensure safe access to the surgical field

Procedures

▶ Burr holes: holes are drilled in the cranium with a neurosurgical drill (craniotome) to relieve a subdural hematoma
▶ Craniotomy for tumor removal: an incision into the cranium to permit access to the brain and intracranial structures. Tumor removal is an indication for a craniotomy
▶ Craniectomy: removal of cranial bone to access the structures below. The bone that is removed is not replaced
▶ Cerebral aneurysm surgery: performed to isolate a cerebral aneurysm from the normal circulation while preserving flow to the nearby vessels
▶ arteriovenous malformation (AVM) resection: performed to correct the fistula that occurs when an abnormal communication exists between the cerebral arteries and veins
▶ Correction of craniosynostosis: performed to correct the premature closure of an infant's cranial suture lines by separating the involved bones and treating the bones to prevent resealing until the brain has completed most of its growth

► Cranioplasty: an area of bone in the skull is replaced with a bone graft or prosthetic material to restore the continuity of the skull, protect the brain, and improve the patient's cosmetic appearance

► Ventriculoperitoneal/ventricular shunt (VP shunt): used to divert the cerebrospinal fluid away from the ventricles of the brain to another location in the body, such as the peritoneal cavity, pleural space, or atrium of the heart, where the cerebrospinal fluid (CSF) can be absorbed

► Transsphenoidal hypophysectomy: performed to remove all or a part of the pituitary gland. The surgical approach is through the sphenoid

► Resection of a vestibular schwannoma (acoustic neuroma): performed to remove tumors from the vestibular branch of cranial nerve VIII while preserving the function of the nerve

► Stereotactic surgery: uses computer-based technology to identify specific structures or lesions in the brain for diagnosis or treatment

► Deep brain stimulation (DBS): performed to change the electrical activity of the brain in a controlled manner using electrodes and a pulse generator

► Endoscopic ventriculoscopy: performed to relieve ventricular obstruction and to restore cerebral spinal circulation, visualization of the third ventricle, decompression, or tissue removal. Stereotactic techniques may be used to improve accuracy

► Microvascular decompression of cranial nerves: Compression of cranial nerves by nearby blood vessels can result in a variety of painful conditions:
  » Trigeminal neuralgia: severe pain in the eyes, lips, nose, scalp, forehead, and jaw
  » Glossopharyngeal neuralgia: pain in the tongue, throat, tonsils, and ear
  » Hemifacial spasm: periodic muscular contractions over one side of the face

► Cerebral revascularization (cerebral bypass): performed to improve the blood flow to an ischemic area of the brain

Spinal Procedures

► Anterior cervical diskectomy and fusion (open): to excise one or more herniated cervical intervertebral disks

► Posterior cervical laminectomy: performed to access the cervical spinal cord and to remove a portion of the cervical lamina

► Application of a halo brace: used to provide traction and restore spinal alignment to the cervical spine. It may also be used to provide initial decompression of the spinal cord after injury

► Lumbar laminectomy and diskectomy: performed to access the lumbar spinal cord and remove a portion of the lumbar lamina. Diskectomy is performed to excise and remove a portion of the intervertebral disk

► Foraminotomy: performed to relieve pressure on the spinal nerves. When the nerves are compressed by bone herniated disk, scarring, or ligament hypertrophy, the patient may experience symptoms of pain, numbness, or weakness in the area served by that particular nerve

► Microdiskectomy: a small window is made in the lamina for access to an intervertebral disk. This is a minimally invasive approach to lumbar laminectomy and diskectomy

► Lumbar fusion: performed to stabilize the spine using a bone graft or metal implant. The graft stimulates the growth of new bone between the vertebral elements, causing the area to fuse. If necessary, metal implants are used to further stabilize the spine and offer greater support

► Correction of scoliosis: performed to restore anatomical alignment to the spine, prevent further curvature, and provide stability

► Spinal tumors: removed surgically to restore circulation of spinal fluid and increase patient mobility and also for pain management

Neurosurgical Pain Management

► Cordotomy (chordotomy): to disable pain-conducting tracts in the spinal cord

► Rhizotomy: performed to selectively sever nerve roots in the spinal cord to relieve pain or symptoms related to neuromuscular conditions

▶ Dorsal column stimulator: used to manage chronic pain. The device generates an electrical impulse that causes a tingling sensation, which alters the perception of pain by the patient

Peripheral Nerve Procedures

▶ Ulnar nerve transposition: to free the ulnar nerve from a groove on the medial epicondyle, thereby restoring function and eliminating desensitization of the affected arm
▶ Peripheral nerve resection and repair: a severed nerve, usually in the hand or forearm, is anastomosed to restore function

Chapter Review Questions

1. Which of the following gases is used to create a pneumoperitoneum?
   A. Carbon monoxide
   B. Oxygen
   C. Nitrous
   D. Carbon dioxide

2. During laparoscopy the intra-abdominal pressure should not exceed
   A. 20 mm Hg.
   B. 15 mm Hg.
   C. 10 mm Hg.
   D. 12 mm Hg.

3. A lower oblique incision is used for which of the following procedures?
   A. Small bowel resection
   B. Open cholecystectomy
   C. Inguinal herniorrhaphy
   D. Splenectomy

4. McBurney's incision is used for
   A. open cholecystectomy.
   B. gastrostomy tube placement.
   C. Nissen fundoplication.
   D. appendectomy.

5. For removal of the gallbladder, which of the following structures are clipped and divided?
   A. Cystic duct and cystic artery
   B. Common bile duct and cystic artery
   C. Cystic duct and hepatic artery
   D. Hepatic duct and hepatic artery

6. Meckel's diverticulum is found in the
   A. esophagus.
   B. pylorus.
   C. ileum.
   D. left colon.

7. A(n) _____ hernia is located within Hesselbach's triangle.
   A. indirect
   B. direct
   C. femoral
   D. umbilical

8. All of the following are breast reconstruction procedures *except*
   A. TRAM.
   B. DIEP.
   C. LEEP.
   D. latissimus dorsi.

9. The term for a face lift is
   A. blepharoplasty.
   B. mentoplasty.
   C. augmentation.
   D. rhytidectomy.

10. A graft that includes epidermis and all of the dermis is
   A. cadaver graft.
   B. porcine graft.
   C. full-thickness graft.
   D. split-thickness graft.

11. The condition of male breast excess is
   A. mentoplasty.
   B. gynecomastia.
   C. mammoplasty.
   D. mastopexy.

12. Ectropion procedure repairs
   A. abnormal inversion of the lower eyelid.
   B. aging eyelids.
   C. drooping lower eyelids.
   D. drooping eyebrow.

13. Decortication of the thoracic cavity is the removal of
   A. a lobe.
   B. the lung.
   C. the parietal pleura.
   D. nodes for biopsy.

14. The procedure performed to correct premature closure of an infant's cranial suture line is
   A. cranioplasty.
   B. craniosynostosis.
   C. ventriculoscopy.
   D. microvascular decompression.

15. The procedure performed to relieve intracranial pressure is
   A. burr holes.
   B. otoplasty.
   C. VP shunt.
   D. stereotactic procedure.

16. Which of the following is not a procedure for chronic pain management?
   A. Chordotomy
   B. Dorsal column stimulator
   C. Cryosurgery
   D. Rhizotomy

17. Which of the following procedures is performed for an incompetent cervical os and to prevent spontaneous abortion?
   A. Shellick
   B. Shirodkar
   C. LEEP
   D. Burch

18. An oophorectomy is the surgical removal of
   A. the fallopian tube and ovary.
   B. the ovum.
   C. the ovary.
   D. an ectopic pregnancy.

19. **A trachelectomy is the removal of**
    A. the uterus.
    B. the cervix.
    C. the endometrium.
    D. the uterine septum.

20. **The removal of one or both testes is a/an**
    A. orchiopexy.
    B. orchiectomy.
    C. varicocelectomy.
    D. vasectomy.

Answers

1. **D.** Carbon dioxide is used to create a pneumoperitoneum in laparoscopy. It is non-flammable and inexpensive and absorbed by the body.
2. **B.** The intra-abdominal pressure should not exceed 15 mm Hg.
3. **C.** The lower oblique incision is used for an inguinal hernia.
4. **D.** McBurney's incision is used for an appendectomy.
5. **A.** The cystic duct and cystic artery are clipped and divided during the cholecystectomy.
6. **C.** Meckel's diverticulum is found in the ileum.
7. **B.** Direct hernia.
8. **C.** LEEP procedure is not a breast reconstruction procedure.
9. **D.** Rhytidectomy is the term for facelift.
10. **C.** Full-thickness skin graft.
11. **B.** Gynecomastia.
12. **C.** Drooping eyelids are repaired with an ectropion procedure.
13. **C.** Removal of the parietal pleura. A surgical removal of restrictive tissue from the visceral pleura. Used to treat entrapped lungs.
14. **B.** Craniosynostosis.
15. **A.** Burr holes.
16. **C.** Cryosurgery is not used to treat chronic pain.
17. **B.** Shirodkar.
18. **C.** The ovary.
19. **B.** Cervix.
20. **B.** Orchiectomy.

References

Archie CL, Roman AS. Normal & abnormal labor & delivery. In DeCherney AH, Nathan L, Laufer N, Roman AS, eds. *CURRENT Diagnosis & Treatment: Obstetrics & Gynecology.* 11th ed. New York, NY: McGraw-Hill; 2013. Retrieved July 25, 2016, from http://accessmedicine.mhmedical.com/content.aspx?bookid=498&Sectionid=41008596.

Barrett KE. Functional anatomy of the liver and biliary system. In Barrett KE, ed. *Gastrointestinal Physiology.* 2nd ed. New York, NY: McGraw-Hill; 2014. Retrieved July 24, 2016, from http://accessmedicine.mhmedical.com/content.aspx?bookid=691&Sectionid=45431411.

Brunicardi F, Andersen DK, Billiar TR, Dunn DL, Hunter JG, Matthews JB, Pollock RE, eds. *Schwartz's Principles of Surgery.* 10th ed. New York, NY: McGraw-Hill Education; 2014.

Butterworth JF IV, Mackey DC, Wasnick JD. Anesthesia for thoracic surgery. In Butterworth JF IV, Mackey DC, Wasnick JD, eds. *Morgan & Mikhail's Clinical Anesthesiology.* 5th ed. New York, NY: McGraw-Hill Education; 2013. Retrieved July 25, 2016, from http://accessmedicine.mhmedical.com/content.aspx?bookid=564&Sectionid=42800557.

Cheng EY, Zarrinpar A, Geller DA, Goss JA, Busuttil RW. Liver. In Brunicardi F, Andersen DK, Billiar TR, Dunn DL, Hunter JG, Matthews JB, Pollock RE, eds. *Schwartz's Principles of Surgery.* 10th ed. New York, NY: McGraw-Hill Education; 2014. Retrieved June 7, 2016, from http://accessmedicine.mhmedical.com/content.aspx?bookid=980&Sectionid=59610873.

Concus AP, Tran TN, Sanfilippo NJ, DeLacure MD. Malignant laryngeal lesions. In Lalwani AK, ed. *CURRENT Diagnosis & Treatment in Otolaryngology—Head & Neck Surgery.* 3rd ed. New York, NY: McGraw-Hill Education; 2011. Retrieved July 25, 2016, from http://accessmedicine.mhmedical.com/content.aspx?bookid=386&Sectionid=39944069.

Cornett PA, Dea TO. Cancer. In Papadakis MA, McPhee SJ, Rabow MW, eds. *CURRENT Medical Diagnosis & Treatment 2016.* New York, NY: McGraw-Hill Education; 2016. Retrieved July 24, 2016, from http://accessmedicine.mhmedical.com/content.aspx?bookid=1585&Sectionid=98107878.

Doherty GM, ed. *CURRENT Diagnosis & Treatment Surgery.* 14th ed. New York, NY: McGraw-Hill Education; 2015.

Fisher WE, Andersen DK, Windsor JA, Saluja AK, Brunicardi F. Pancreas. In Brunicardi F, Andersen DK, Billiar TR, Dunn DL, Hunter JG, Matthews JB, Pollock RE, eds. *Schwartz's Principles of Surgery.* 10th ed. New York, NY: McGraw-Hill Education; 2014. Retrieved July 24, 2016, from http://accessmedicine.mhmedical.com/content.aspx?bookid–980&Sectionid=59610875

Fuller JK. *Surgical Technology Principles and Practice.* 6th ed. Philadelphia, PA: Saunders; 2012.

Gruessner AC, Jie T, Papas K, Porubsky M, Rana A, Smith M, Yost SE, Dunn D, Gruessner RG. Transplantation. In Brunicardi F, Andersen DK, Billiar TR, Dunn DL, Hunter JG, Matthews JB, Pollock RE, eds. *Schwartz's Principles of Surgery.* 10th ed. New York, NY: McGraw-Hill Education; 2014. Retrieved July 24, 2016, from http://accessmedicine.mhmedical.com/content.aspx?bookid=980&Sectionid=59610852.

Jobe BA, Hunter JG, Watson DI. Esophagus and diaphragmatic hernia. In Brunicardi F, Andersen DK, Billiar TR, Dunn DL, Hunter JG, Matthews JB, Pollock RE, eds. *Schwartz's Principles of Surgery.* 10th ed. New York, NY: McGraw-Hill Education; 2014. Retrieved July 24, 2016, from http://accessmedicine.mhmedical.com/content.aspx?bookid=980&Sectionid=59610867.

Kim EJ, Maas CS. Blepharoplasty. In Lalwani AK, ed. *CURRENT Diagnosis & Treatment in Otolaryngology—Head & Neck Surgery.* 3rd ed. New York, NY: McGraw-Hill Education; 2011. Retrieved May 22, 2016, from http://accessmedicine.mhmedical.com/content.aspx?bookid=386&Sectionid=39944121

Kitagawa Y, Dempsey DT. Stomach. In Brunicardi F, Andersen DK, Billiar TR, Dunn DL, Hunter JG, Matthews JB, Pollock RE, eds. *Schwartz's Principles of Surgery.* 10th ed. New York, NY: McGraw-Hill Education; 2014. Retrieved July 24, 2016, from http://accessmedicine.mhmedical.com/content.aspx?bookid=980&Sectionid=59610868.

Konety BR, Carroll PR. Urothelial carcinoma: cancers of the bladder, ureter, & renal pelvis. In McAninch JW, Lue TF, eds. *Smith and Tanagho's General Urology.* 18th ed. New York, NY: McGraw-Hill Education; 2012. Retrieved July 24, 2016, from http://accessmedicine.mhmedical.com/content.aspx?bookid=508&Sectionid=41088098.

Lal G, Clark OH. Thyroid, parathyroid, and adrenal. In Brunicardi F, Andersen DK, Billiar TR, Dunn DL, Hunter JG, Matthews JB, Pollock RE, eds. *Schwartz's Principles of Surgery.* 10th ed. New York, NY: McGraw-Hill Education; 2014. Retrieved July 24, 2016, from http://accessmedicine.mhmedical.com/content.aspx?bookid=980&Sectionid=59610880.

Lalwani AK, ed. *CURRENT Diagnosis & Treatment in Otolaryngology—Head & Neck Surgery.* 3rd ed. New York, NY: McGraw-Hill Education; 2011.

LeBlond RF, Brown DD, Suneja M, Szot JF (2015). Nonregional Systems and Diseases. In LeBlond RF, Brown DD, Suneja M, Szot JF, eds. *DeGowin's Diagnostic Examination.* 10th ed. New York, NY: McGraw-Hill Education; 2014. Retrieved July 25, 2016, from http://accessmedicine.mhmedical.com/content.aspx?bookid=1192&Sectionid=68665331.

Lee GA, Masharani U. Disorders of the thyroid gland. In Lalwani AK, ed. *CURRENT Diagnosis & Treatment in Otolaryngology—Head & Neck Surgery.* 3rd ed. New York, NY: McGraw-Hill Education; 2011. Retrieved May 31, 2016, from http://accessmedicine.mhmedical.com/content.aspx?bookid=386&Sectionid=39944082.

Leventhal D.D., Constantinides M. Rhinoplasty. In Lalwani AK, ed. *CURRENT Diagnosis & Treatment in Otolaryngology—Head & Neck Surgery.* 3rd ed. New York, NY: McGraw-Hill Education; 2011. Retrieved May 22, 2016, from http://accessmedicine.mhmedical.com/content.aspx?bookid=386&Sectionid=39944122.

Liang MK, Andersson RE, Jaffe BM, Berger DH. The appendix. In Brunicardi F, Andersen DK, Billiar TR, Dunn DL, Hunter JG, Matthews JB, Pollock RE, eds. *Schwartz's Principles of Surgery.* 10th ed. New York, NY: McGraw-Hill Education; 2015. Retrieved June 07, 2016, from http://accessmedicine.mhmedical.com/content.aspx?bookid=980&Sectionid=59610872.

Mandpe AH. Neck neoplasms & neck dissection. In Lalwani AK, ed. *CURRENT Diagnosis & Treatment in Otolaryngology—Head & Neck Surgery.* 3rd ed. New York, NY: McGraw-Hill Education; 2011. Retrieved July 25, 2016, from http://accessmedicine.mhmedical.com/content.aspx?bookid=386&Sectionid=39944065.

McAninch JW. Disorders of the penis & male urethra. In McAninch JW, Lue TF, eds. *Smith and Tanagho's General Urology.* 18th ed. New York, NY: McGraw-Hill Education; 2012. Retrieved July 24, 2016, from http://accessmedicine.mhmedical.com/content.aspx?bookid=508&Sectionid=41088118.

McAninch JW, Lue TF, eds. *Smith and Tanagho's General Urology.* 18th ed. New York, NY: McGraw-Hill Education; 2012.

Morton DA, Foreman KB, Albertine KH. *Gross Anatomy: The Big Picture.* New York, NY: McGraw-Hill Education; 2011.

Murr AH. Maxillofacial trauma. In Lalwani AK, ed. *CURRENT Diagnosis & Treatment in Otolaryngology—Head & Neck Surgery.* 3rd ed. New York, NY: McGraw-Hill Education; 2011. Retrieved July 24, 2016, from http://accessmedicine.mhmedical.com/content.aspx?bookid=386&Sectionid=39944040.

Pham TH, Hunter JG. Gallbladder and the extrahepatic biliary system. In Brunicardi F, Andersen DK, Billiar TR, Dunn DL, Hunter JG, Matthews JB, Pollock RE, eds. *Schwartz's Principles of Surgery.* 10th ed. New York, NY: McGraw-Hill Education; 2014. Retrieved May 31, 2016, from http://accessmedicine.mhmedical.com/content.aspx?bookid=980&Sectionid=59610874.

Shah SB, Emanuel IA. Nonallergic & allergic rhinitis. In Lalwani AK, ed. *CURRENT Diagnosis & Treatment in Otolaryngology—Head & Neck Surgery.* 3rd ed. New York, NY: McGraw-Hill Education; 2011. Retrieved July 25, 2016, from http://accessmedicine.mhmedical.com/content.aspx?bookid=386&Sectionid=39944047.

Stoller ML. Retrograde instrumentation of the urinary tract. In McAninch JW, Lue TF, eds. *Smith and Tanagho's General Urology.* 18th ed. New York, NY: McGraw-Hill Education; 2012. Retrieved July 24, 2016, from http://accessmedicine.mhmedical.com/content.aspx?bookid=508&Sectionid=41088088.

Suh JD, Chiu AG. Acute & chronic sinusitis. In Lalwani AK, ed. *CURRENT Diagnosis & Treatment in Otolaryngology—Head & Neck Surgery.* 3rd ed. New York, NY: McGraw-Hill Education; 2011. Retrieved July 25, 2016, from http://accessmedicine.mhmedical.com/content.aspx?bookid=386&Sectionid=39944049.

Vasconez HC, Buseman J. Plastic & reconstructive surgery. In Doherty GM, ed. *CURRENT Diagnosis & Treatment Surgery.* 14th ed. New York, NY: McGraw-Hill Education; 2015. Retrieved July 25, 2016, from http://accessmedicine.mhmedical.com/content.aspx?bookid=1202&Sectionid=71528355.

Welch KC, Goldberg AN. Sleep disorders. In Lalwani AK, ed. *CURRENT Diagnosis & Treatment in Otolaryngology—Head & Neck Surgery.* 3rd ed. New York, NY: McGraw-Hill Education; 2011. Retrieved July 25, 2016, from http://accessmedicine.mhmedical.com/content.aspx?bookid=386&Sectionid=39944080.

Wolf JS Jr, Stoller M. Laparoscopic surgery. In McAninch JW, Lue TF, eds. *Smith and Tanagho's General Urology.* 18th ed. New York, NY: McGraw-Hill Education; 2012. Retrieved July 24, 2016, from http://accessmedicine.mhmedical.com/content.aspx?bookid=508&Sectionid=41088086.

Zoumalan R, Leventhal D, White W. The aging face: Rhytidectomy, browlift, midface lift. In Lalwani AK, ed. *CURRENT Diagnosis & Treatment in Otolaryngology—Head & Neck Surgery.* 3rd ed. New York, NY: McGraw-Hill Education; 2011. Retrieved May 22, 2016, from http://accessmedicine.mhmedical.com/content.aspx?bookid=386&Sectionid=39944120.

14

Patient Monitoring and Medical Emergencies

PHYSIOLOGICAL MONITORING DURING SURGERY

In a state of well-being, the body responds readily to stimuli to maintain life. Many complex biochemical, physical, and metabolic processes control the balance between stimuli and responses. Examples are shivering (uncontrollable muscle tremor) when the body's temperature drops and vasoconstriction (constriction of blood vessels) when blood pressure falls. This maintenance of physiological balance is called homeostasis.

Physiological monitoring is assessment of the patients vital metabolic functions. All anesthetics (regional, general, or sedative) require physiological monitoring. However, the complexity and type of monitoring depend on the type of anesthesia, the patient's physical condition, the known risks, and the anticipated complications

▶ Monitoring Devices and Use:
  » Pulse oximetry: blood oxygen saturation and heart rate
  » Automatic blood pressure cuff: blood pressure
  » Electrocardiography: heart rhythm; heart rate; myocardial ischemia
  » Capnography: adequacy of ventilation; airway pressure
  » Oxygen analyzer: delivered oxygen concentration
  » Ventilator pressure monitor: ventilator disconnection during general anesthesia and assisted ventilation; monitor airway pressure
  » Temperature monitoring probe (Foley type): core body temperature
  » Urine output using Foley catheter: gross indication of renal perfusion and intravascular volume
  » Central venous catheter: measures central venous pressure; rapid administration of fluids and blood; drug administration
  » Arterial catheter: measurement of arterial blood pressure; obtain samples of arterial blood for analysis
  » Precordial Doppler: detects air embolism
  » Transesophageal echocardiography: to evaluate myocardium; assess valve function; assess intravascular volume; detection of air embolism
  » Esophageal Doppler: assessment of descending aortic flow; assessment of cardiac preload
  » Transpulmonary indicator dilution: cardiac output; cardiac preload
  » Esophageal and precordial stethoscope: auscultation of breathing and heart sounds
▶ Monitoring process: The standards of monitoring patients are set by the American Society of Anesthesiologists (ASA). The routine parameters that must be monitored include the following:
  » Oxygenation
  » Ventilation
  » Cardiac function

    » Perfusion

    » Body temperature

    » Neuromuscular response

    » Fluid and electrolyte balance

▶ Pulmonary ventilation is the total mechanism for drawing air into the lungs. Perfusion is the movement of oxygenated blood to the peripheral capillaries where oxygen is exchanged for carbon dioxide at the cellular level

    » Capnography: the partial pressure of expired carbon dioxide

    » Arterial blood gas (ABG): blood gases are measured using a sample of arterial blood

    » Pulse oximeter: a digital sensor that detects oxygen saturation in the hemoglobin by spectrometry

▶ Fluid and electrolyte balance

    » Electrolyte balance is measured by a blood test, and fluid volume is indicated by arterial blood pressure and blood loss. Blood loss is calculated during surgery by measuring the amount of total fluids (blood and irrigation fluid) suctioned from the wound and subtracting the total amount of irrigation fluids used. Blood loss is also estimated by weighing surgical sponges. (**Note:** This is why it is so important for the surgical technologist to keep track of the amount of irrigation fluid the surgeon uses during a case.)

▶ Circulatory function and perfusion

    » Circulatory assessment includes monitoring of heart function and peripheral circulation

        • Direct monitoring requires the insertion of a measuring device (e.g., internal pulmonary artery catheter) inside the patient's body

    » Electrocardiography (ECG): measures the electrical activity of the heart, which is projected into a waveform

    » Arterial blood pressure monitoring: blood pressure is measured manually with a sphygmomanometer and blood pressure cuff or automatically using a digital blood pressure monitoring system

    » Transesophageal monitoring: a transesophageal stethoscope may be used to monitor the heart's rhythm, intensity, pitch, and frequency during general anesthesia

    » Intravascular monitoring: hemodynamic monitoring is used to measure central venous pressure, mean artery pressure, stroke volume, and cardiac output

    » Pulmonary artery catheter (PAC): used for critical care monitoring in selected patients

▶ Renal function

    » Kidney function can be grossly measured by observing renal output during surgery. More specific tests such as blood urea nitrogen (BUN) are used to measure substances in the blood that are not effectively filtered by the kidneys

▶ Body temperature

    » The normal body temperature is 97° to 99.5°F (36° to 37.5°C). The body can tolerate environmental temperatures outside this range, but only with protection. The core temperature must be maintained within a range compatible with life. (**Note:** For irrigation into a body cavity, it is very important for the surgical technologist to use saline that is not too hot for internal organs.)

DELIBERATE HYPOTHERMIA

▶ Deliberate hypothermia (lowering of the patient's core body temperature) is used during malignant hyperthermia. This is a physiological reaction to specific anesthetics and neuromuscular blocking agents in which the body temperature is critically elevated

    » Blood may be diverted to a cooling system

    » IV administration of a cold solution and irrigation of body cavities with a cold fluid

    » Saline ice slush is packed around the heart to produce localized cooling in cardiac surgery

    » Target temperatures are no lower than 78.8°F (26°C)

NEUROMUSCULAR RESPONSE

▶ During general anesthesia, neuromuscular blocking agents are administered to relax skeletal muscles. Without adequate muscle relaxation or paralysis, retraction of the body wall and other tissues is difficult, and this prevents adequate exposure of the operative site. A peripheral nerve stimulator is used to monitor the level of neuromuscular blocking.

LEVEL OF CONSCIOUSNESS

▶ The patient's level of consciousness is monitored to prevent intraoperative awareness (IOA). This is a rare phenomenon in which the patient retains some degree of consciousness (including sensory awareness) but lacks motor ability. The bispectral index system (BIS) is used to prevent patient recall of pain perceived during surgery. Although intraoperative awareness is rare, the psychological consequences are serious and include posttraumatic symptoms.

MONITORING MEDICAL EMERGENCIES

▶ Advanced Trauma Life Support (ATLS)
  » The clinical problem that is the most lethal (the greatest threat to life) is addressed first
  » Treatment is initiated even when a definitive diagnosis (a diagnosis confirmed by assessment of investigation) is not established
  » Treatment may be initiated even when there is no detailed history
▶ The Golden Hour
  » Refers to the first critical hour following injury
  » Trauma-related morbidity and mortality are partially related to the time elapsed between the trauma event and resuscitation attempts
  » About 50% of victims with injury to the aorta, heart, spinal cord, or brainstem die from their injuries within minutes of the trauma
  » A further 30% of victims die in the first few hours
  » Of these, half will have died from hemorrhage and the remaining from damage to the central nervous system. Overall, hemorrhage is the primary cause of death in traumatic injury

Chapter Review Questions

1. **What is measures blood oxygen saturation and heart rate?**
   A. Oxygen analyzer
   B. Pulse oximetry
   C. Capnography
   D. Oxygen analyzer

2. **What is the *Golden Hour*?**
   A. The time it takes to turn over a surgical suite after a surgical procedure
   B. How long the patient is in the postanesthesia care unit
   C. The first critical hour following an injury
   D. The time it takes to get to an emergency room

3. **What percentages of victims with injury to the aorta, heart, spinal cord, or brainstem die from their injuries within minutes of the trauma?**
   A. 30%
   B. 40%
   C. 50%
   D. 60%

4. **What is used to prevent patient recall of pain perceived during surgery?**
   A. BIS
   B. ECG
   C. EEG
   D. GIA

5. **What is used to monitor the level of neuromuscular blocking?**
   A. Pulse oximetry
   B. PAC
   C. BUN
   D. Peripheral nerve stimulator

6. **How is blood loss measured during a surgical procedure?**
   A. Anesthesia personnel keeps track of all IVs given
   B. Surgical technologist keeps track of irrigation on the field
   C. Circulator weighs the laps and sponges
   D. All of the selections are correct

7. **What is the lowest temperature a patient can be taken to for hypothermia?**
   A. 80.2°F (25°C)
   B. 78.8°F (26°C)
   C. 79°F (20°C)
   D. 68.8°F (26.2°C)

8. **What is used to measure substances in the blood that are not effectively filtered by the kidneys?**
   A. BUN
   B. ATLS
   C. PAC
   D. ASA

9. **What is intraoperative awareness?**
    A. When a patient is able to speak to the surgical team during a surgical procedure
    B. When a patient raises their arm in the middle of a surgical procedure
    C. When the patient retains some degree of consciousness (including sensory awareness) but lacks motor ability
    D. When the patient is under local anesthesia and moves all extremities when they feel pain

10. **What is a physiological reaction to specific anesthetics and neuromuscular blocking agents in which the body temperature is critically elevated?**
    A. Hypothermia
    B. Malignant hyperthermia
    C. Hyperthermia
    D. Malignant hypothermia

Answers

1. **B.** A Pulse Oximetry measures blood oxygen saturation and heart rate.
2. **C.** The first critical hour following an injury is the "Golden Hour".
3. **A.** 30% of victims with injury to the aorta, heart, spinal cord, or brainstem die from their injuries within minutes of the trauma.
4. **A.** The Bispectral Index System (BIS) is used to prevent patient recall of pain perceived during surgery.
5. **D.** A peripheral nerve stimulator is used to monitor the level of neuromuscular blocking.
6. **D.** Blood loss is measured during a surgical procedure using the following methods: anesthesia personnel keeps track of all IVs given; surgical technologist keeps track of irrigation on the field; circulator weighs the laps and sponges used.
7. **B.** The lowest temperature a patient can be taken to for Hypothermia is 78.8°F (26°C).
8. **A.** Blood Urea Nitrogen (BUN) is used to measure substances in the blood that are not effectively filtered by the kidneys.
9. **C.** When the patient retains some degree of consciousness (including sensory awareness) but lacks motor ability, this is called "intraoperative awareness".
10. **B.** Malignant hyperthermia is a physiological reaction to specific anesthetics and neuromuscular blocking agents in which the body temperature is critically elevated.

Reference

Fuller J. *Surgical Technology: Principles and Practice.* 6th ed. Philadelphia, PA: Saunders.

Postoperative Procedures

15

Patient Transportation and Specimens

SAFE TRANSPORTATION OF THE PATIENT
Transportation of the patient is the responsibility of all perioperative team members.

Transport to the OR
The surgical technologist may assist in the transportation of the surgical patient to the operating room (OR) when not in the scrubbed role. Procedures to follow when transporting patients to the OR include:

- Review of patient name, room number, and special considerations with the charge nurse prior to transport
- Identify oneself and purpose at the nursing unit
- Confirm patient's identification bracelet and procedure with the patient and nurse by asking the patient to state their name, date of birth, and other information on the bracelet. Procedural information can be confirmed at this time
- When transporting a patient via stretcher, ensure that both side rails are up and locked
- Ensure all devices are secure to stretcher: IVs, oxygen, and drainage devices
- Cover patient with blankets
- Transport patients on stretchers feet first, slowly, ensuring hands and feet are within the rails
- For patients on stretchers, enter elevator head first. Back wheelchair in to elevator so patient is facing forward
- Patients should be brought to a holding area and never left alone. Inform patients of where they are and introduce them to the new care provider

Transfer
- Patient assessment is required to determine the amount of assistance the patient will require to move to the OR bed
  - » Patients have been medicated and my not be able to follow commands or may not be able to move easily because of the effects of medication
- A minimum number of four (4) perioperative personnel are needed to transfer a patient from a stretcher to the OR bed for patient and perioperative staff safety
  - » One at the head, one on either side of the patient, and one at the foot
- The same number of personnel (4) are needed to transfer the patient to the stretcher upon completion of the procedure
- Care should be used not to shear the skin when transferring by using sheets as a mode of transfer
- Transfer devices designed to assist in the transfer of patients eliminate skin and tissue injury along with personnel injury
  - » Roller

The holding or preoperative area is where patients are prepared for surgery. The chart is reviewed and a preoperative physical assessment is performed.

» Slider board
» HoverMatt air mattress
▶ Procedure for transfer (pre-procedure)
» Move stretcher close to the OR bed with the side rail down against the OR bed
» Lock the stretcher (the person on the side of the stretcher stabilizes the stretcher in the locked position)
» Personnel are positioned on each side of the patient, one at the head and one at the foot
  • For a mobile and awake patient, a perioperative member at each side of the patient may be sufficient
» If possible, have the patient move to the OR bed and position themselves in a position of comfort
  • Be mindful of the IV and any other tubing during transfer
» Secure the patient safety strap before moving the stretcher
» Once the patient is secured, unlock the stretcher remove it from the OR
▶ Once patient is transferred onto the OR bed, a pillow is placed under the patient's head and a safety strap is placed 2 inches above the knees for a standard supine position
» A pillow may be placed under the patient's knees for comfort
» The safety strap and patient position may be altered after the induction of anesthesia, depending on the surgical site
» The patient's arms may be positioned on arm boards at no more than 90 degrees abduction to prevent nerve damage and secured with safety straps
» Compression boots/stockings are connected prior to the induction of anesthesia
» A warming blanket of forced hot air may also be used

Postprocedure Transfer

▶ Do not move the patient without the consent of the anesthesia provider
▶ Have all equipment and personnel available prior to move
▶ Use a designated system, such as counting ("on 3") to indicate when the move will begin
▶ Use proper body mechanics at all times

SPECIMENS

A minimum of four perioperative team members is needed for safe transfer of a patient postoperatively or one who is medicated.

Specimen handling and identification is defined by each institution in its hospital pathology policy. The surgical technologist should be familiar with the policy and review the procedures for specimen protocol.

Specimens are collected from the patient during the surgical procedure.

Types of Specimens

▶ Organ
▶ Tissue sample
▶ Body fluid
▶ Foreign body or material
▶ Blood
▶ Bone

Care and Handling of Specimens

▶ When specimens are anticipated, sterile containers should be available on the sterile field to keep handling to a minimum or to avoid handling (such as portion of bowel or infected tissue)
▶ Specimen handed from the surgeon to the surgical technologist is confirmed immediately as a specimen and the name repeated aloud for the circulating nurse for verification
▶ The name of the specimen or a letter can be written down on a sterile label to identify the specimen in a container on the sterile field until it can be handed off to the circulator

▶ Sutures may be used for orientation purposes and should be noted by all team members aloud and recorded for verification
  » "short" = superior
  » "long" = lateral
▶ The specimen remains on the surgical field until the circulator is prepared to accept the specimen and the surgeon gives permission to pass off the specimen from the surgical field
▶ The specimen is verified by all members of the surgical team when the specimen is passed off the surgical field
▶ A counted sponge is never used to pass off a specimen from the sterile field. (A counted sponge could be inadvertently placed in a specimen container, resulting in an incorrect sponge count.)
▶ The specimen is verified as
  » Type of specimen; such as origin
  » Laterality if applicable
  » Required laboratory tests
  » Specific handling procedures required
▶ All information should be confirmed via the "read back" method with the surgical technologist and circulator
▶ The specimen is placed in a labeled pathology container for transport to pathology and documented on the pathology request by the circulator
▶ The type of preservative is determined by the study requested by the surgeon and the pathology department
▶ Routine specimens may be sent in formaldehyde (10% formalin) for permanent section
▶ Specimens are recorded on the pathology request and in the patient record
▶ The number and names of the specimens are verified by the surgical team

Special Specimen Procedures

▶ Amputated limbs: sent to pathology or to morgue in an impervious wrap and bag. Some religious beliefs require the limb to be buried
▶ Breast tissue: sent for immediate examination for estrogen and progesterone receptor sites without preservative
▶ Body fluids: sent for immediate examination. Collected in a Lukens trap (bronchial, peritoneal)
▶ Calculi and teeth: gallstones, ureteral. Sent without preservative and no fluid
▶ Cultures: anaerobic or aerobic culture of fluid or tissue. Sent immediately to the lab
▶ Cytology: for cell studies. These are often placed on a slide and secured with a fixative. May be sent to the lab via swab
▶ Frozen sections: for identification of malignancy or immediate tissue identification. No solution or preservative, may be moistened with saline solution
▶ Foreign bodies: an object that has been introduced into the body that does not belong in the body, such as a prosthesis or a retained surgical item. These objects may be examined grossly.
▶ Product of conception (embryo/fetus): often determined by hospital policy. This specimen may require chromosomal/genetic testing at a laboratory outside of the hospital.

DEFINITIONS

Biopsy: removal of tissue for laboratory examination.

Cultures: growth of cells or microorganisms in a growth medium. Cultures can be aerobic or anaerobic.

Frozen section: thin cross-section of a frozen specimen used for microscopic diagnosis.

Gram stain: method of staining that differentiates bacteria by the chemical composition of the cell walls.

Gross examination: examination of a specimen without the aid of magnifying instruments. (Example: gross exam of teeth or hardware removed.)

Chapter Review Questions

1. All of the following assist in patient transfer and eliminate skin and tissue damage *except*
   A. HoverMatt air mattress.
   B. roller.
   C. sheet.
   D. slider board.

2. The surgical specimen is passed off the surgical field when
   A. the surgical technologist receives the specimen.
   B. the surgeon gives permission and the circulator is ready to receive the specimen.
   C. the surgeon gives permission and the surgical technologist agrees to pass it off.
   D. the entire team agrees to pass off the specimen.

3. When transporting a patient to the operating room, the surgical technologist should
   A. push the stretcher from the foot when entering the operating room.
   B. pull the stretcher using the IV pole.
   C. pull the stretcher by the foot when going into the elevator.
   D. push the stretcher from the head when traveling in the hallways.

4. A specimen for permanent section is usually sent in which of the following solutions?
   A. Sterile saline solution
   B. Sterile water
   C. Formaldehyde (10% formalin)
   D. Methylene blue

5. All of the following are examples of a foreign body specimen *except*
   A. Bullet.
   B. Retained surgical sponge.
   C. Tooth.

6. Orthopedic hardware: The reason the patient's arms are positioned on arm boards not to exceed a 90-degree angle is to prevent injury to
   A. abductor plexus.
   B. brachial plexus.
   C. ulnar nerve.
   D. cervicothoracic nerve.

7. Which one of the following is a vital safety consideration involved in patient transfer?
   A. Ensuring that the patient has warm blankets
   B. Ensuring that the stretcher is locked
   C. Ensuring that the patient has DVT stockings on
   D. Ensuring that the surgeon is in the room to identify the patient

8. The surgeon is performing an exploratory laparotomy. She wants to do pelvic washings. The surgical technologist knows that he will need a _____ to collect the fluid for the specimen.
   A. sterile specimen cup
   B. Lukens trap
   C. culture tube
   D. sterile basin

9. ST Anne Marie is asked to bring Mrs. Jones to the preoperative holding room from the waiting room one floor away. Mrs. Jones is in a wheelchair. Anne Marie knows that she should:
   A. push the wheelchair in head first into the elevator and back out of the elevator.
   B. back the wheelchair in to the elevator so the patient is facing forward.
   C. go in head first with the wheelchair and turn so she can exit facing forward.
   D. transfer the patient to a stretcher.

10. All of the following are sent to the laboratory for specimen without fixative *except*
   A. renal calculi.
   B. breast tissue for frozen section.
   C. gallstones.
   D. appendix.

Answers

1. **C.** The use of a sheet as a mode of transfer can shear the skin when transferring a patient.
2. **B.** The surgeon must give permission to pass off the specimen, and the circulator must be ready to receive the specimen so it is properly labeled.
3. **D.** The stretcher should be pushed by the head to avoid injury and for safe transport of the patient.
4. **C.** Formaldehyde (10% formalin).
5. **C.** A tooth is not a foreign body. It is found in the body naturally.
6. **B.** The brachial plexus would be stressed if extended past 90 degrees and lead to nerve damage.
7. **B.** Ensuring the stretcher is locked is a vital safety concern for the patient.
8. **B.** A Lukens trap is attached to the suction to allow for fluid to be collected and sent for specimen.
9. **B.** When transporting a patient by wheelchair, back into the elevator so the patient is facing forward.
10. **D.** The appendix would be sent with formalin. All others would be sent without a fixative.

References

Booth, K. Stoia, J. *Anatomy, Physiology & Disease for the Health Professions*. 3rd ed. New York: McGraw-Hill; 2013.

McAdam AJ, Onderdonk AB. Laboratory Diagnosis of Infectious Diseases. In Kasper D, Fauci A, Hauser S, Longo D, Jameson J, Loscalzo J, eds. *Harrison's Principles of Internal Medicine*. 19th ed. New York, NY: McGraw-Hill Education; 2015. Retrieved June 26, 2016, from http://accessmedicine.mhmedical.com/content.aspx?bookid=1130& Sectionid=63652694.

Medical Dictionary for Allied Health McGraw Hill.

16

Contaminated Waste and Room Turnover

During a surgical procedure in the operating room, many times the patient's body fluids will get on the surfaces of the equipment, floor, walls, and personnel. It is important to make sure all traces of the patient are removed from all surfaces of the room before you bring the next patient in for their procedure. You do not want to cross-contaminate the surgical suite. The floor is wet-vacuumed or mopped to loosen all soil and debris and remove it completely. Perioperative staff put on clean scrub attire, which is put on at the start of each day and is changed whenever it becomes soiled or wet.

▶ Contamination: The consequence of physical contact between a sterile surface and a nonsterile surface in surgery. Contamination also can result from airborne dust, moisture droplets, or fluids that act as a vehicle for transporting contaminants from a nonsterile surface to a sterile one
▶ Waste: The by-product of something (i.e., the wrapper of an item or the hair that fell while brushing your hair); something not needed after a process has taken place
▶ Decontamination: a process in which instruments and supplies are first cleaned and then processed through chemical or mechanical means so that they are safe for handling
▶ Disinfection: a process that removes most but not all microbes on inanimate (nonliving) surfaces. Some disinfectants are formulated for use on surgical equipment, whereas others are used for environmental cleaning
▶ Cleaning: the process of removing surface soil, blood, body fluids, and other kinds of organic debris, usually with detergents and mechanical action (scrubbing or washing)
▶ Bacteriostatic: refers to an agent that inhibits bacterial colonization (growth) but does not destroy bacteria
▶ Antisepsis: a process that greatly reduces the number of microorganisms on skin or other tissue
▶ Bactericidal: able to kill bacteria

ENVIRONMENTAL DISINFECTANTS

Environmental disinfectants are used for routine low-level disinfection and terminal decontamination. These disinfectants contain enzymes and other chemicals that destroy or inhibit microbes by changing cell proteins (denaturation) or by drying them (desiccation). The Material Safety Data Sheet (MSDS) describes the formulation, safe use, precautions, and emergency response for all chemicals used in the workplace. This is usually kept at the front desk of the surgery department.

▶ Phenolics: Phenol (carbolic acid) if formulated as a detergent for hospital cleaning
▶ Quaternary ammonium compounds (quats): are fungicidal and bactericidal but not effective at killing spores
▶ Hypochlorite: is sporicidal and tuberculocidal and effective against the human immunodeficiency virus (HIV). The Centers for Disease Control and Prevention (CDC) recommends this product for use in spot cleaning of blood spills, because it is very fast acting

▶ Alcohol: a commonly used disinfectant that is composed of two components: ethyl alcohol and isopropyl alcohol. Alcohol is not sporicidal, but it is bactericidal, tuberculocidal, and virucidal.

INTRAOPERATIVE ROUTINE

▶ During surgery, the circulator and his/her assistants are responsible for ensuring that the environment in the surgical suite is kept as disease-free as possible
  » Any blood spills or contamination by other organic material should be removed promptly with a hospital-grade disinfectant
  » All articles used and discarded in the course of surgery must be placed in leak-proof containers
  » Any contaminated or suspect item must be handled in a manner that protects personnel from contamination
  » Tissue specimens, blood, and all other body fluids must be placed in a leak-proof container for transport out of the department
  » Because paper products are difficult or impossible to decontaminate, every effort should be made to keep patients' charts, laboratory slips, radiography reports and radiographs, and any paper documentation free of contamination
  » Contaminated sponges must be collected in a kick bucket in which a plastic bag or liner has been previously placed
  » Instruments that fall off the surgical field must be retrieved by the circulator (with gloves protecting the hands) and placed in a basin containing a noncorrosive disinfectant
  » During surgery, the surgical technologist should periodically wipe blood and tissue from instruments
  » Small-bore cannulas and suction tip lumens should be flushed frequently to prevent interior buildup of debris
  » Any organic debris or residue that remains is a potential source of pathogenic microorganisms, even if the item has been through the sterilization or disinfection process

POSTOPERATIVE SEQUENCE

▶ The patient is transferred out of the operating room in stable condition
▶ Surgical instruments and supplies are sorted and prepared for decontamination
▶ All disposable items are placed in designated containers
▶ Documentation is completed and signed off (circulator and surgical technologist)
▶ Soiled instruments and reusable supplies are transported to the decontamination area
▶ Specimens are documented and transported to a designated area for pickup
▶ The surgical suite is cleaned and decontaminated for the next case
  » All trash and linen are taken out of the room
    • Trash that has come in contact with the patient's bodily fluids is separated for proper disposal
  » All surfaces are wiped down with an antibacterial cleaning solution
  » The floors are cleaned with a cleaning solution that is acceptable for the surgical environment to effectively kill all microorganisms that may be present in the room (**Note:** No new supplies are allowed to be brought into the room until the floors have been properly cleaned.)
  » The linen is put back on the bed and clean trash liners are put back in place (**Note:** anesthesia equipment is cleaned as well.)
▶ Equipment and furniture are returned to their normal locations

Chapter Review Questions

1. **What is disinfection?**
   A. Destruction of microorganisms by heat or chemical means
   B. Ability to kill germs (bacteria)
   C. A chemical that breaks down organic debris by emulsification
   D. Nonliving

2. **Which one is *not* an environmental disinfectant?**
   A. Hypochlorite
   B. Alcohol
   C. Saline
   D. Quaternary ammonium compounds

3. **What is done at the beginning of the day before the start of the first surgical case in the operating room?**
   A. Damp dusting of surgical lights, furniture, and fixed equipment in the operating suite
   B. Furniture is placed in its normal position
   C. Clean surgical attire is put on by personnel
   D. All of the above

4. **During a surgical procedure, what must be done to prevent cross-contamination with blood-borne pathogens?**
   A. Soiled linen must be removed from operating table
   B. Any blood spills or contamination by other organic material should be removed promptly with a hospital-grade disinfectant
   C. All disposable anesthesia equipment is removed in closed bags
   D. Clean linen and liner bags are placed on bed and in trash frames

5. **Which disinfectant is effective against the HIV virus?**
   A. Phenol
   B. Quaternary ammonium compounds
   C. Saline
   D. Hypochlorite

6. **Which one is part of the postoperative routine to clean a surgical suite?**
   A. Damp dust surgical lights
   B. All contaminated items used during the cleaning process are removed from the room
   C. Contaminated sponges must be collected in a kick bucket
   D. All of these things are don postoperatively

7. **What are the two components that make up alcohol?**
   A. Ethyl and isopropyl
   B. Hypochlorite and ammonium
   C. Ethyl and phenol
   D. Ammonium and isopropyl

8. **When doing a room turnover, when should you bring your new supplies into the room to start opening for your next case?**
   A. As soon as the patient is taken out of the room
   B. As soon as the patient is brought into the room
   C. As soon as the trash and soiled linen is taken out of the room
   D. As soon as the floor has been mopped after all surfaces have been disinfected

9. **If an instrument falls on the floor during a surgical procedure, what must be done with the instrument?**
    A. The circulator puts the instrument back on the sterile field
    B. The surgical technologist picks it up and puts it on the back table
    C. The circulator picks it up, with gloved hand, and puts it in a basin containing a disinfectant
    D. The surgical technologist resterilizes the instrument and puts it back on the sterile field

10. **Can tissue that has been left on an instrument ever be considered sterile?**
    A. Yes
    B. No
    C. Only if the instrument was put in the autoclave to be sterilized
    D. Only if the sterile instrument was packed separately from the instrument set in a peel pack

Answers

1. **A.** Disinfection is the destruction of microorganisms by heat or chemical means.
2. **C.** Saline is NOT an environmental disinfectant. It can cause instruments to have "pits".
3. **D.** At the beginning of the day before the start of the first surgical case in the operating room, damp dusting of surgical lights, furniture, and fixed equipment in the operating suite; furniture is placed in its normal position; and clean surgical attire is put on by personnel.
4. **B.** Any blood spills or contamination by other organic material should be removed promptly with a hospital-grade disinfectant during a surgical procedure to prevent cross-contamination with blood-borne pathogens.
5. **D.** Hypochlorite disinfectant is effective against the HIV virus.
6. **B.** All contaminated items used during the cleaning process are removed from the room which is part of the postoperative routine to clean a surgical suite.
7. **A.** The two components that make up alcohol is Hypochlorite and ammonium.
8. **D.** As soon as the floor has been mopped after all surfaces have been disinfected, then you can bring your new supplies into the room to start opening for your next case in a room turnover.
9. **C.** If an instrument falls on the floor during a surgical procedure, the circulator picks it up, with gloved hand, and puts it in a basin containing a disinfectant.
10. **B.** No tissue left on an instrument can ever be considered sterile.

Reference

Fuller J. *Surgical Technology: Principles and Practice*. 6th ed. Philadelphia, PA: Saunders.

Administrative Requirements

17

Patient Documentation

PATIENT CHARTING

The patient's chart is used to document information pertinent to the care of the patient. This can be an electronic medical record (EMR) or a worksheet used prior to final documentation, such as a count sheet.

The patient's medical record in paper or electronic form may contain:

► Identification of the patient
  » Name, date of birth, patient identification number
► History and physical exam, including medical history
► Medications
► Allergies
► Admitting diagnosis
► Physician orders
► Plan of care
► Physical findings and notes from all care providers
► Laboratory test results
► Surgical consent (see Chapter 5)
► Discharge plan
► Follow-up instruction and treatment plan

THE PERIOPERATIVE RECORD

The perioperative record is often referred to as the intraoperative record. It is the documentation for the patient from the time the patient enters the operating room until the time of discharge to the postanesthesia care unit (PACU).

Documentation on the perioperative/intraoperative record may include:

► Patient's name and date
► Procedure(s)
► Surgeon(s)
► Surgical team members
  » Anesthesia care provider
  » Perioperative nurse
  » Surgical technologist
  » Surgical assistant
  » Other
    • Students
    • Sales representative
► Patient's physical status
► Type of anesthesia administered
► Patient's emotional status and level of consciousness upon arrival and discharge from operating room

- ▶ Patient assessment preoperative, intraoperative, and postoperative
- ▶ Surgical skin antisepsis used
- ▶ Surgical skin clips used
- ▶ Patient position and devices used
- ▶ Position of safety strap
- ▶ Catheters and drain placement
- ▶ Implants
- ▶ The Time Out procedure
- ▶ Incision or start of procedure
- ▶ End of procedure
- ▶ Surgical counts
  - » The type of count—instrument, sponge, suture
  - » Outcome—e.g., correct
  - » Surgical team members participating in the surgical count
- ▶ Specimen documentation
- ▶ Medications and fluids administered from the sterile field
- ▶ Patient skin assessment pre- and postoperative
- ▶ Surgical wound classification
- ▶ Equipment
  - » ESU and pad placement

THE SURGEON'S PREFERENCE CARD

The preference card is a list of instrumentation, supplies, and equipment a surgeon requires to perform a specific procedure. The list is maintained and updated by perioperative nurses and is regarded as a physician's order. The preference card is reviewed by the surgeon. Such items as medication are reviewed prior to the surgical procedure.

The preference card can contain

- ▶ Patient position
- ▶ Medication
- ▶ Surgical room configuration
- ▶ Specimen information
- ▶ Procedural information
- ▶ Instrument sets
- ▶ Suture
- ▶ Equipment
- ▶ Drapes and draping procedures

SURGICAL COUNTS

Surgical counts are the key to patient safety and a priority for the surgical team. Retention of a surgical item can have catastrophic effects for the patient and is a preventable event.

Surgical counts are performed:

- ▶ Prior to the patient entering the room
- ▶ Without interruption
- ▶ Audibly, concurrently, and visually by both the RN circulator and ST in the scrub role
- ▶ Prior to the start of the procedure
- ▶ When there is a change in perioperative team members (RN circulator and the ST in the scrub role) such as shift change or meal break
- ▶ At the request of any team member
- ▶ When items are added to the initial count
- ▶ When wound closure is initiated
- ▶ Before the closure of a cavity within a cavity
- ▶ At closure of fascia
- ▶ At skin closure or when items are no longer in use
- ▶ In accordance to institutional policy

The initial count is:

- ▶ Performed when all items are opened prior to the incision being made and patient entering the operating room

► Used as a baseline count
► Performed and documented by two perioperative personnel: the circulating nurse and the surgical technologist in the scrub role

The first closing count is:

► Performed at the beginning of the closure of peritoneum or the first layer of any cavity
► An additional count is required for procedures with a cavity within a cavity such as a cesarean section. (The additional count begins at the start of closure of the uterus.)

The second closing count is:

► Performed at the beginning of the closure of fascia or the layer before subcutaneous

The final closing count:

► Is performed as soon as the closure of skin is initiated or at the end of the procedure when counted items are no longer in use
► Begins with the sterile field, the Mayo stand, back table, and the items discarded from the surgical field (such as sponges in bag counters or dropped instruments)

In case of an incorrect count:

► The surgeon must be notified immediately of an incorrect count
► No further closing procedures may take place until the lost item is found or incorrect count is rectified
► All team members must participate in locating the lost item
► Repeat the count
► Notify the charge nurse
► X-ray the surgical site
► All actions taken are documented if the item is not located

Precautions for counted items:

► Counted items should never leave the OR during the surgical procedure
► Only radiopaque soft goods must be used on the sterile field
  » Soft goods include:
    • Lap sponges and packs
    • Raytec sponges
    • Kittner or peanut dissector
    • Cottonoid patties
  » When counting soft goods/sponges they must be separated and counted aloud and be visible to both the ST (scrub person) and RN circulator
  » The band is removed once the package is counted
  » A package containing an incorrect number of soft goods (such as 9 or 4) is removed from the sterile field and bagged and marked. These items are not included in the count.
► All sutures are counted upon opening packages to verify the presence of needle(s)
► Keep a minimum number of counted sponges on the sterile field
► Note aloud the number of packs in the abdomen to the perioperative team and when packs are removed
► Secure all sharps in needle counters
► Exchange suture needles on a one-for-one basis
► Account for all broken items: instruments, sutures, blades
► Do not accept dressing sponges until after the final count is performed
► Other items in the surgical count include (but not limited to):
  » Suture reels
  » Suture boots/shods
  » Umbilical tapes
  » Vessel loops
  » Hypodermic needles
  » Free needles
  » Rulers
  » Marking pens

Chapter Review Questions

1. The initial surgical count is performed
   A. prior to the use of instruments.
   B. after the Time Out.
   C. prior to incision.
   D. when items are added to the sterile field.

2. The patient's medical record documents includes which of the following?
   A. History and physical exam
   B. Medications
   C. Discharge plan
   D. Surgical consent
   E. All of the above

3. The perioperative patient record documents all of the following *except*
   A. surgical counts.
   B. surgical team members.
   C. surgical wound classification.
   D. surgeon's preference card.

4. Which of the following team members perform the surgical count?
   A. The surgical technologist and the surgeon
   B. The surgical technologist and the RN circulator
   C. The surgical technologist and the first assistant
   D. The surgeon and the RN circulator

5. During the surgical count a laparotomy sponge is unaccounted for. The first action taken is to
   A. call for x-ray.
   B. notify the supervisor.
   C. recount the sponges.
   D. notify the surgeon.

6. Surgical counts are performed
   A. prior to the start of the procedure.
   B. when an item is added to the initial count.
   C. when the anesthesia provider is relieved.
   D. when wound closure is initiated.
      i.   A, B, & C
      ii. B, C, & D
      iii. A, B, & D

7. Which of the following is the correct statement about surgical counts?
   A. The RN circulator can count items on the back table while the ST in the scrub role is busy with the closure
   B. To save time, the dressing sponges can be accepted by the ST prior to the final count
   C. Counted items should never leave the OR during a surgical procedure
   D. Broken instruments should be removed from the field and discarded in the trash to avoid receiving them back in the tray

8. What is the correct order in which a surgical count is performed at closing?
   A. Items off the field, back table, Mayo stand, sterile field
   B. Sterile field, Mayo stand, back table, items off the field
   C. Mayo, back table, items off field, sterile field
   D. Back table, Mayo, sterile field, items off the sterile field

9. Counted items include all of the following *except*
    A. sponges.
    B. vessel loops.
    C. medicine cups.
    D. hypodermic needles.

10. **When counting a pack of laparotomy sponges during the initial count, if only 4 sponges are noted, the correct action is to**
    A. ask for another pack and take one to make up the difference.
    B. have the difference noted on the count sheet.
    C. hand off the sponges and have them contained and labeled.
    D. place the sponges aside on the back table and do not use them.

Answers

1. **C.** The initial surgical count is performed prior to incision.
2. **E.** All of the items are documented on the patient's medical record.
3. **D.** The surgeon's preference card is not documented on the perioperative record.
4. **B.** The surgical technologist and the RN circulator.
5. **D.** Notify the surgeon. After notifying the surgeon a recount can be performed.
6. **D. iii.** A, B, & D
7. **C.** Counted items should never leave the OR during a surgical procedure.
8. **B.** Sterile field, Mayo stand, back table, items off the field.
9. **C.** Medicine cups.
10. **C.** Hand off the sponges and have them contained and labeled.

References

Frey KB, Ross T. *Surgical Technology for the Surgical Technologist, A Positive Care Approach.* 4th ed. New York, NY: Delmar; 2014.

Goodman T, Spry C. Prevention of retained surgical items. In *Essentials of Perioperative Nursing.* 6th ed. Burlington, MA: Jones & Bartlet Publisher; 2017.

18

Computer Technology

COMPUTERS IN THE PERIOPERATIVE ENVIRONMENT

▶ Computer technology is incorporated into many different types of equipment and biomedical devices used in the perioperative environment:
  » Secure computer systems for recording patient information (patient charts) and other medical records
  » Preference cards for surgeons
  » Diagnostic imaging equipment
  » Digital cameras and image output on monitors (screens) during surgical procedures
  » Robotic surgical systems
  » Computer tracking of hospital supplies, instruments, and equipment during reprocessing
  » Automatic patient billing systems for supplies used in surgery
  » Computerized operation of sterilizers and instrument decontamination equipment

HOW COMPUTERS WORK

▶ The computer's main function is to store data and retrieve those using electrical signals. The data are stored on chips, or small electrical circuits that are not readily visible

COMPUTER TERMS AND LANGUAGE

▶ What the computer does (e.g., displaying an email)
▶ The equipment needed to perform the tasks
▶ The process used to make the equipment work
▶ Electronic information is called data
▶ Pictures on a computer screen are called images
▶ The process of entering information into the computer (by humans or another machine) is called inputting
▶ Information received from the computer is called output

HARDWARE (PHYSICAL COMPONENTS)

▶ The core unit contains the wiring and complex circuits that run the computer and store data
▶ The peripherals are other types of equipment that interface with the computer and are part of its operation, such as the computer screen, keyboard, and mouse
  » Central processing unit (CPU): the computer memory and electronic components that enable programming and output
  » Memory (RAM, random access memory): this connects with the main electrical circuits to perform all the tasks needed to operate the computer
  » Motherboard: the primary circuits that run the computer

- » Drive: internal or external device that stores the computer's data
- » Monitor: the computer's screen where data are viewed by the user
- » Modem/wireless card: an electronic device that makes transmissions to or from a computer via a communication line
- » Keyboard: alphanumeric device for inputting data to the computer
- » Mouse: the user's steering component for inputting data on the monitor
- » Speakers: provide sound output from the computer
- » Hard copy: computer output that has been reproduced in the form of a CD, DVD, or paper printout
- » Printer/scanner/fax: output and input devices that produce paper and electronic documentation
- » USB port: a type of serial port for connecting peripheral devices to a computer system
- ▶ Computer software:
  - » The term *software* is used to describe programs that control the tasks a computer can perform. The computer needs instructions from the software to perform the tasks that individuals require it to do
- ▶ Operating system: The OS is the electronic controller of all the data the computer needs to perform tasks. The most common operating systems are Microsoft Windows, Mac OS, and Linux systems.
- ▶ Computer programs: perform specific tasks. An application is used to produce text documents, calculate mathematical equations, play music, or display photographs
  - » Word processing: performs the functions of a typewriter with many additional features
  - » Database or spreadsheet: allows the user to enter complex data involving items, lists, and numerical or arithmetic information
  - » Graphic design: provides the computing tools needed to "draw" and manipulate figures or to create complex images based on quantitative data
  - » Interactive educational programs: designed to help the user learn subjects such as mathematics, languages, and physical sciences

BASIC COMPUTER USE

- ▶ Computer motor skills
  - » Typing skills are required to enter data into the computer quickly and with minimum of errors
  - » Operation of the mouse
- ▶ Elementary operations
  - » Start: the computer begins to boot up
  - » Desktop: the background for all computer programs
  - » Files and folders: an electronic location where data are stored
  - » Window: a rectangular frame that displays the boundaries of a document, graphic, or other image on the monitor
  - » Toolbar: located at the top of a window
  - » Menu: list of optional commands the user can select while viewing or manipulating data
  - » Scrolling: method used to "turn pages" on the computer screen
- ▶ Word processing
  - » Creating a document
  - » Formatting text
    - • Font
    - • Changing case
    - • Indents and spacing
    - • Page numbers
    - • Selecting and changing text
    - • Editing text: delete, move, paste text, spell check
    - • Graphics
    - • Saving data
    - • Printing documents

COMPUTER NETWORKS

▶ Types of networks: the term *computer network* refers to two or more computers that are connected electronically. Networks allow the transfer of information from one computer to another.
  » Internet: vast computer network; the World Wide Web is part of the Internet
  » Intranet: a system of multiple computers within a facility or organization that allows communication only within that system
▶ Navigating the Internet and World Wide Web
  » Internet search
    • Open the Internet browser installed on the computer by clicking on it
    • Look for the address bar in the Internet toolbar
    • Enter http://www.google.com in the address bar and click OK or Go to confirm
    • Enter the search topic in the search box. Click on any of the search results to access the information
    • Once you have accessed the pertinent information, you can add this reference site to your Favorites in your Internet browser for future reference
  » Email: this process allows individuals or groups to contact each other through email programs on a network or the Internet and to send and receive messages, documents, and graphics electronically. Healthcare institutions often set up email systems for their employees as a means of communicating messages and sending documents

KEY CONCEPTS

▶ The relationship between medicine and modern technology is one of increasing interdependence
▶ Health care workers and providers are now challenged to balance the use of technology with the human side of medicine
▶ The study of physics is fundamental to understanding the technological aspects of medicine
▶ Computer technology is now an integral part of many medical devices and is also a common method of documentation and communication in health care facilities
▶ The most basic components of the computer include the central processing unit, keyboard, mouse, and monitor
▶ Health facilities use a computer network system or intranet to allow communication and access to important data by employees

Chapter Review Questions

1. What is a CPU?
   A. A compilation of information, usually lists or numerical information, that can be manipulated or calculated
   B. The component of a computer that contains the circuitry, memory, and power controls
   C. Data storage devices that are an integral part of the computer
   D. A computer network within a facility or an organization that can be accessed only by those employed or affiliated with the organization

2. Which one of these is *not* a way to incorporate computer technology in the perioperative environment?
   A. Recording patient information and other medical records
   B. Preference cards
   C. Diagnostic imaging equipment
   D. Informing the patient in ICU of their condition

3. What is considered hardware?
   A. Spreadsheet
   B. Graphic design
   C. Monitor
   D. Word processing

4. What is the user's steering component for inputting data on the monitor?
   A. Keyboard
   B. Speakers
   C. Mouse
   D. USB port

5. What is electronic information called?
   A. Data
   B. Images
   C. Inputting
   D. Output

6. What are interactive educational programs?
   A. Programs that provides the computing tools needed to "draw" and manipulate figures
   B. Programs that are designed to help the user learn different subjects
   C. Programs that allows the user to enter complex data involving items, lists, and numerical information
   D. Programs that perform the functions of a typewriter with many additional features

7. How would you find a list of optional commands the user can select while viewing or manipulating data?
   A. Use the toolbar
   B. Scroll through the page
   C. Look where the data is stored
   D. Use the menu

8. What can you use to analyze the spelling and grammar of the text?
   A. Spell check
   B. Graphics
   C. Formatting text
   D. None of the above

9. **If you are going to communicate with your co-workers in your hospital and you do not want anyone outside the hospital system to see the message, what electronic system would you use to communicate with them?**
   A. World Wide Web
   B. Intranet
   C. Office mail
   D. Fax

10. **What is data computer output that has been reproduced in the form of a CD, DVD, or paper printout?**
    A. Modem/wireless card
    B. Motherboard
    C. Hard copy
    D. Printer/scanner/fax

Answers

1. **B.** A CPU is the component of a computer that contains the circuitry, memory, and power controls.
2. **D.** Recording patient information and other medical records; preference cards; diagnostic imaging equipment are all ways to incorporate computer technology in the perioperative environment.
3. **C.** A monitor is considered to be hardware.
4. **C.** A mouse is the user's steering component for inputting data on the monitor.
5. **A.** Electronic information is called "Data".
6. **B.** Programs that are designed to help the user learn different subjects are interactive educational programs.
7. **D.** You would find a list of optional commands the user can select while viewing or manipulating data by using the menu.
8. **A.** Spell check is used to analyze the spelling and grammar of the text.
9. **B.** You would use the Intranet if you are going to communicate with your co-workers in your hospital and you do not want anyone outside the hospital system to see the message.
10. **C.** A hard copy is data computer output that has been reproduced in the form of a CD, DVD, or paper printout.

Reference

Fuller J. *Surgical Technology: Principles and Practice.* 6th ed. Philadelphia, PA: Saunders.

19

Environmental Safety and All Hazards Preparedness

Risk is the statistical probability of a harmful event; it is defined as the number of harmful events that occur in a given population over a stated period. Risk and probability are not difficult to measure when sentinel event reporting is performed each time there is an accident or injury in the workplace.

SAFETY STANDARDS AND RECOMMENDATIONS

▶ ECRI Institute: nonprofit research organization designated as an evidence-based practice center: http://www.ecri.org
▶ Association for Professionals in Infection Control and Epidemiology (APIC): http://www.apic.org
▶ U.S. Environmental Protection Agency (EPA): http://www.epa.gov
▶ U.S. Food and Drug Administration (FDA): http://www.fda.gov
▶ The Joint Commission: http://www.jointcommission.org
▶ Occupational Safety and Health Administration (OSHA): http://www.osha.gov

TECHNICAL RISKS

Fire Risks

All accredited health care facilities have a responsibility and mandate to orient employees and students to fire safety practices, including the use of fire extinguishers and facility evacuation procedures.

▶ Fire triangle:
  » Oxygen (available in the air or as a pure gas)
  » Fuel (a combustible material)
  » Source of ignition (usually in the form of heat)
▶ Flammable chemicals
  » Alcohol is now commonly used in skin prep solutions and is a high-risk source of fuel in surgical fires
▶ Medical devices
  » Rubber, plastic, Silastic, and vinyl materials are flammable
  » Disposable anesthesia equipment, such as endotracheal tubes, airways, masks, cannulas, and corrugated tubing, is a hazardous source of fuel
▶ Drapes and gowns
  » Surgical drapes and gowns are flame resistant; however, in an OEA (Oxygen Enriched Area) they can ignite easily
  » The operating table mattress and positioning devices made of foam and liquid gels also are potential fuel

▶ Intestinal gases
  » The intestine normally produces hydrogen, oxygen, nitrogen, carbon dioxide, and methane
  » Methane is explosive at concentrations of 5% to 15%
▶ Sources of ignition: any heat-producing device has the potential to cause a fire
  » Laser: approximately 13% of surgical fires involve lasers
  » Electrosurgical unit (ESU): the active electrode can reach 1292°F (700°C), hot enough to ignite surgical drapes and other supplies
  » High-speed instruments: when high-speed drills are used, the active tip is irrigated to prevent the buildup of heat created by friction between the metal tip and the bone
  » High-intensity light: the light source is delivered through a fiberoptic cable. When the cable is detached from the endoscope, light emitted from the cable can easily ignite drapes, cloth, or other materials
  » Electrical malfunction: an electrical short or other malfunction can cause sparking (electrical arching), which can ignite combustible materials on the surgical field
▶ Fires in the operating room
  » Patient fire: approximately 21% of patient fires occur in the airway, 44% on the face, 8% inside the patient, and 26% on the skin. There are three steps that are immediately taken to protect the patient and stop the fire:
    • Shut off the flow of all gases to the patient's airway
    • Remove any burning objects from the surgical site
    • Assess the patient for injury and respond appropriately
  » Structural fire: RACE
    • Rescue patients in the immediate area of the fire
    • Alert other people to the fire
    • Contain the fire
    • Evacuate personnel

Electricity

▶ Risk: electrical malfunctions are a leading cause of hospital fires in the United States
▶ Electrical energy:
  » Current: the rate of electrical (electron) flow
  » Voltage: the driving force behind the moving electrons
  » Impedance (resistance): the ability of a substance to stop the flow of electrons (electricity)
  » Grounding: the discharge of electrical current from the source to ground

Ionizing Radiation

▶ Radiograph machines, fluoroscopes, and unshielded radioactive implants produce ionizing radiation in amounts high enough to damage tissue

Magnetic Resonance Imaging (MRI)

▶ Whenever MRI is used, the primary risk is the presence of metal, which can be drawn from its source and into the path of the powerful magnetic field

Chemical Risks

▶ Toxic chemicals
  » The majority of the different kinds of hazardous chemicals can produce serious long-term effects, such as respiratory or skin problems, genetic changes, and fetal injury
  » It is important to remember that although exposure to a particular chemical may be brief, constant exposure to chemicals in a variety of work situations has a cumulative effect
▶ Smoke plume
  » This is created during laser surgery and electrosurgery

» Smoke plumes contain harmful toxins that must be removed from the immediate surgical environment because they are known to contain benzene, hydrogen cyanide, formaldehyde, blood fragments, and viruses—potentially harmful when inhaled
  • Always suction the smoke (plume) while using the bovie. Surgical personnel have been known to develop polyps in the nostrils from the plume side box note

BIOLOGICAL RISKS

▶ Disease transmission in the perioperative environment
  » The primary focus of disease control in the health care environment is on preventing contact with blood and body fluids
▶ Standard Precautions: The practices of the standard apply to all patients and all contact with blood and body fluids
  » Personal protective equipment (PPE)
  » Hand hygiene and asepsis
  » The special handling of biological waste and linens
  » Special handling procedures for sharp items
  » Specific procedures when a health care worker is injured by a contaminated needle or other sharp
  » Disinfection (decontamination) of all inanimate surfaces in the medical environment
  » Decontamination of all medical devices and instruments between patients
  » Encouraging single-use medical supplies and equipment when possible
▶ Sharps injury
  » Sharps are such a threat to health care personnel that OSHA has issued the Blood-Borne Pathogen Rule, a special set of regulations for handling and disposing of sharps
▶ Human factor
  » Working too quickly
  » Distraction from the task at hand
  » Failure to comply with precautions and standards
  » Extreme fatigue
  » Distraction related to environmental noise, including loud music and conversation
  » Lack of support in designing and maintaining a prevention program
  » Difficulty abandoning old and valued methods of working
  » Difficulty adapting to newer, safer medical devices
▶ Postexposure prophylaxis (PEP)
  » A risk reduction strategy that is used after exposure to blood or other body fluids
▶ Transmission-based precautions
  » Are implemented when a patient is known or suspected to have a highly infectious disease and Standard Precautions are insufficient to prevent transmission to others
▶ Hazardous waste
  » The Environmental Protection Agency (EPA) defines medical waste as any solid waste generated in the diagnosis, treatment, or immunization of humans or animals, in research that involves people or animals, or in the production or testing of biological waste
    • Soiled or blood-soaked bandages
    • Culture dishes and other glassware
    • Discarded surgical gloves after surgery
    • Needles used to give injections or draw blood
    • Cultures, stocks, and swabs used to inoculate cultures
    • Removed body organs
▶ Latex Allergy
  » True allergy to latex rubber is a risk to patients and personnel. True allergy is differentiated from other types of immune responses

MUSCULOSKELETAL RISKS

▶ Causes of musculoskeletal injury
  » Exertion: the amount of physical effort needed to perform a task
  » Posture: twisting or turning the body disrupts normal balance

» Repetitive motion: places stress on tendons and muscles.

» Contact stress: excessive direct pressure against a sharp edge or hard surface

▶ Mechanical injury prevention in the environment

» In the operating room, musculoskeletal injuries most often occur as a result of the following:

- Lifting, positioning, transporting, and transferring the patient
- Retrieving and shelving heavy instrument trays overhead or near the floor
- Moving heavy equipment
- Catching items that are falling
- Tripping over tubing or electrical cords
- Balancing a heavy instrument tray in the hand while distributing it onto the sterile field
- Attaching cords to wall sockets or overhead inline connectors
- Climbing over operating room clutter or trying to retrieve a heavy item from a cluttered environment

Chapter Review Questions

1. **What is personal protective equipment (PPE)?**
   A. Clothing or equipment that protects the wearer from direct contact with hazardous chemicals or potentially infectious body fluids
   B. Agents or substances capable of supporting a fire
   C. Exposure to hazardous chemicals or contact with potentially infected blood and body fluids
   D. A cell-mediated immune response to a substance in the body

2. **Which one of these is *not* an agency that creates and make recommendations about injury in the health care setting?**
   A. APIC
   B. EPA
   C. FDA
   D. AORN

3. **What is considered a source of fuel for a fire in the operating room?**
   A. Alcohol
   B. Drapes and gowns
   C. Intestinal gases
   D. All of the above

4. **What is *voltage*?**
   A. The rate of electrical flow
   B. The driving force behind the moving electrons
   C. The ability of a substance to stop the flow of electrons
   D. The discharge of electrical current from the source to ground

5. **Why is an MRI a risk in the medical environment?**
   A. It uses ionizing radiation in amounts high enough to damage tissue
   B. It can cause serious long-term effects, such as respiratory or skin problems
   C. The presence of metal
   D. It contains harmful toxins that must be removed from the immediate surgical environment

6. **All are Standard Precautions *except***
   A. PPE.
   B. hand hygiene.
   C. recapping needles.
   D. decontamination.

7. **Which one of the following is a human factor for risk of injury in the operating room?**
   A. Difficulty abandoning old and valued methods of working
   B. Retractable or self-sheathing needles
   C. Mounting and removing a blade with an instrument
   D. None of the above

8. **What is *hazardous waste*?**
   A. A cell-mediated immune response to a substance in the body
   B. Any solid waste generated in the diagnosis, treatment, or immunization of humans or animals
   C. A naturally occurring sap obtained from rubber trees that is used in the manufacture of medical devices
   D. The statistical probability of a given event based on the number of such events that have already occurred in a defined population

9. **What can cause a musculoskeletal injury in the medical environment?**
   A. Pushing a cart down the hall
   B. Lifting an object close to the body
   C. Using abdominal muscles to hold the weight of your upper body
   D. Climbing over operating room clutter

10. **What is PEP?**
   A. A risk reduction strategy that is used after exposure to blood or other body fluids
   B. Implemented with a patient is known or suspected to have a highly infectious disease and Standard Precautions are insufficient to prevent transmission to others
   C. The most common means of transmission of blood-borne pathogens to health care workers
   D. A set of practices for handling blood and body fluids

Answers

1. **A.** Personal Protective Equipment is clothing or equipment that protects the wearer from direct contact with hazardous chemicals or potentially infectious body fluids.
2. **D.** AORN is NOT an agency that creates and makes recommendations about injury in the health care setting.
3. **D.** Alcohol drapes and gowns and intestinal gases are all sources of fuel for a fire in the operating room.
4. **B.** The driving force behind the moving electrons is voltage.
5. **C.** The presence of metal in an MRI is a risk in the medical environment.
6. **C.** PPE, hand hygiene and decontamination are all standard precautions.
7. **A.** Difficulty abandoning old and valued methods of working is a human factor for risk of injury in the operating room.
8. **B.** Hazardous Waste is any solid waste generated in the diagnosis, treatment, or immunization of humans or animals.
9. **D.** Climbing over operating room clutter can cause a musculoskeletal injury I the medical environment. Even though all answers are correct, this answer is the best because it causes the worst injury.
10. **A.** PEP is a risk reduction strategy that is used after exposure to blood or other body fluids.

Reference
Fuller J. *Surgical Technology: Principles and Practice.* 6th ed. Philadelphia, PA: Saunders.

Index

Note: Page number followed by f and t indicates figure and table respectively.